Lone Parent Families

Pearson
Education

We work with leading authors to develop the
strongest educational materials in sociology,
bringing cutting-edge thinking and best learning
practice to a global market.

Under a range of well-known imprints, including
Prentice Hall, we craft high-quality
print and electronic publications which help
readers to understand and apply their content,
whether studying or at work.

To find out more about the complete range of our
publishing please visit us on the World Wide Web at:
www.pearsoneduc.com

Lone Parent Families

Gender, Class and State

Karen Rowlingson
and
Stephen McKay

An imprint of **Pearson Education**

Harlow, England · London · New York · Reading, Massachusetts · San Francisco · Toronto · Don Mills, Ontario · Sydney
Tokyo · Singapore · Hong Kong · Seoul · Taipei · Cape Town · Madrid · Mexico City · Amsterdam · Munich · Paris · Milan

Pearson Education Limited
Edinburgh Gate
Harlow
Essex CM20 2JE

and Associated Companies throughout the world.

Visit us on the World Wide Web at:
www.pearsoneduc.com

First published in Great Britain in 2002

ISBN 0 582 28761 8

British Library Cataloguing-in-Publication Data
A catalogue record for this book is available from the British Library

10 9 8 7 6 5 4 3 2

Library of Congress Cataloging-in-Publication Data
A catalog record for this book is available from the Library of Congress

08   07   06   05   04   03   02

Typeset by 35 in 9/13.5 pt Stone Serif
Printed in Malaysia

contents

introduction

Lone parenthood is now a central issue in social policy and in the sociology of the family. There have been many books that are relevant to lone
parenthood but very few of these have tried to give an overview of the
context, the policy issues and the large number of research studies that
have investigated different dimensions of lone parenthood. This book
aims to provide such an overview. The book is aimed at students of social
policy/administration, sociology, social studies, social work and gender/
women's studies. It will also be of interest to academics and professionals
in these fields.

The title of the book illustrates the main subject matter and the main
themes of the book. We are interested in lone parent families including
the lone parent, the child or children in the family and the non-resident
parent. Nine out of ten lone parents are lone mothers and gender is a key
factor affecting most aspects of lone parenthood. But gender is not the
only key factor in the lives of lone parent families. In Britain, most lone
parents are from working class backgrounds and this aspect of their lives
can also help to explain the creation of lone parent families and also their
experiences. The final theme throughout the book is the role of the state.
We argue that the British state makes policy towards lone parents under
the influence of capitalist and patriarchal assumptions. Sometimes these
influences are contradictory – it may be in the interests of capitalism for
lone parents to engage in the labour market whereas patriarchal interests
may be better served if women stay in the home. These influences are
therefore not straightforward and they are by no means the only imperatives guiding social policy, but they are important forces that need to be
investigated.

The book is in two parts. The first considers the context surrounding lone parenthood. After providing a profile of lone parent families today the section takes a broader historical look at lone parenthood. Various theoretical perspectives and definitional issues are tackled in Chapter 3 before Part One ends with a chapter devoted to investigating the role of the state in this field. Part Two of the book considers, in turn, particular areas of social policy including poverty and social security, work and employment, the care and welfare of children, non-resident parents and maintenance, and health, housing and hardship. Part Two ends where it began, with evidence of the great poverty and hardship experienced by lone parent families. A concluding chapter expands on the main themes of the book.

In writing this book, we have received help from, and would therefore like to thank, a number of people, including Jo Campling (as consultant editor), Matthew Smith and Liz Tarrant (at Pearson Education) and Jane Millar (at the University of Bath). We would also like to thank colleagues (past and present) at the Policy Studies Institute (PSI). The PSI has carried out a series of surveys of lone parent families since 1991 and we draw heavily on the data from these surveys. We would like to thank our colleagues for producing such excellent material that tells us so much about lone parent families. We have also enjoyed working with them in an environment that is sometimes frenetic but mostly fun.

Crown copyright is reproduced with the permission of the Controller of Her Majesty's Stationery Office.

We would also like to thank all the lone parents who have taken part in these studies. Without their co-operation we would never have been able to write this book.

And finally we would like to thank our own parents, to whom this book is dedicated. Having recently become parents ourselves, we appreciate what a difficult job it is and so wish to thank them for their love and support throughout our lives.

Karen Rowlingson   Stephen McKay
Lecturer in Social Research   Principal Research Fellow
University of Bath   Policy Studies Institute

March 2001

list of figures

list of tables

list of boxes

acknowledgements

We are grateful to the following for permission to reproduce copyright material:

Table 1.5 from *Absent Fathers* by Bradshaw *et al.* published by Routledge, 1999; Table 6.4 from *Lone Parents, Employment and Social Policy: Cross-National Comparisons* edited by Millar and Rowlingson, published by The Policy Press, 2001; Figure 6.1 from *Making Work Pay* by Bryson *et al.*, published by The Joseph Rowntree Foundation, 1997; and Box 3.1 from *Lone Mothers, Paid Work and Gendered Moral Rationalities* edited by S. Duncan and R. Edwards, published by Palgrave Publishers Ltd, 1999. Crown copyright material is reproduced under Class Licence number CO1 W0000039 with the permission of the Controller of HMSO and the Queen's Printer for Scotland.

Whilst every effort has been made to trace the owners of copyright material, in a few cases this has proved impossible and we take this opportunity to offer our apologies to any copyright holders whose rights we may have unwittingly infringed.

part one

The context

In Britain today, one family in four is a lone parent family and one child in three will spend part of their childhood in a lone parent family. Lone parent families have been the subject of intense interest, whether because of concern about their poverty or the welfare of their children or the costs to the tax-payer. This book discusses the recent growth of lone parent-hood and the social policy implications of this growth. In a field where myth often impedes reality, let us begin with a few key facts:

Box 1   Key facts about lone parenthood

- The number of lone parent families in Britain tripled from about half a million in the early 1970s to over 1.5 million in the mid-1990s – including 2.7 million children (Haskey 1998).

- About one-quarter of all families with children were headed by a lone parent in the late 1990s (Department of Social Security 2000).

- Compared with the rest of Europe, Britain has a very high rate of lone parenthood, a very high rate of teenage pregnancy and a very high rate of divorce (Bradshaw *et al.* 1996).

- Lone parent families are one of the poorest groups in British society today, and most receive means-tested benefits of one kind or another (Department of Social Security 2000).

- About nine in ten lone parents are women (Marsh *et al.* 2001).

- Women from working class backgrounds are more likely than others to become lone parents (own analysis of the *Family and Working Lives Survey* 1994–95; see Appendix 1).

This part of the book sets the scene for the discussion of the more specific social policy issues in Part Two.

Chapter 1 gives an overview of the numbers and characteristics of lone parents in Britain today. It points out that families change through time and this means that few children spend their entire childhoods continuously as part of a lone parent family. This chapter also places British lone parents in an international context. For example, the USA has a much higher rate of lone parenthood than Britain which in turn has one of the highest rates in Europe (with many of the Scandinavian countries close behind).

One of the reasons for interest in lone parenthood is that there has been a rapid growth in the number of lone parent families in recent years. The statistics behind this growth are given in Chapter 2 along with a discussion of possible explanations. But Chapter 2 also places the recent growth of lone parenthood into a broader historical context to argue that lone parent families have been on the scene for centuries. The low rate of lone parenthood in the 1950s and 1960s is perhaps at least as striking, in historical terms, as the higher rate of lone parenthood in more recent years. Having said this, the growth in numbers of never-married single mothers may be a peculiarly recent development.

A number of theoretical perspectives on lone parenthood are explored in Chapter 3 before it is argued that lone parent families must be understood in terms of both their class and gender position within society. A section on 'approaches to parenthood and childhood' reminds us that such concepts should not be taken for granted in our consideration of lone parent families. Contemporary norms around parenthood and childhood inevitably affect the way we see lone parenthood and the way that policies are designed in relation to them. The chapter concludes by explaining how, despite their widespread use, the terms 'lone parent' and 'single mother' are actually quite difficult to define, and that family life is rather more complex than can be captured by very simple definitions.

Chapter 4 considers the role of the state in relation to lone parenthood. Once again, concepts of class and gender are pertinent here. The chapter discusses the role of the state in 'private life' and focuses on two particular areas of private life: the right to reproduction; and the relationships between children and their parents. The chapter concludes by looking at current government policy in relation to family life.

chapter 1

Lone parent families today

1.1 Numbers, characteristics and dynamics

Lone parent families today are a mainstream family type – they are not uncommon. According to the *Households Below Average Income* (see Appendix 1 for further details about data sources on lone parent families) for 1998/99, 8 per cent of all individuals, of all ages, were in lone parent families (Department of Social Security 2000, Table B1). If we just look at families with children, lone parent families made up about one in four of all families with children in 1998/99 (Department of Social Security 2000).

There are well over one-and-a-half million lone parent families in Britain today and around one in four children currently live in a lone parent family (a total of about 3.0 million children: Department of Social Security 2000). But children do not usually live in a lone parent family for the whole of their childhoods – they usually spend only part of their lives in a lone parent family. And about half of those who become lone parents will no longer be so within six years, as we show later in this chapter (Rowlingson and McKay 1998). In 1990, it was estimated that about half of all children would have experienced life in a lone parent family by the year 2000 (Kiernan and Wicks 1990). And there have been similar estimates in the US (American Research Council 1989).

Box 1.1 A mainstream family type

- There are over one-and-a-half million lone parent families in Britain (Haskey 1998).

- Lone parents make up one in four of all families with children (Department of Social Security 2000).

- About three million children currently live in lone parent families (Department of Social Security 2000).

- Approaching half of all children will spend some time in a lone parent family while growing up (Kiernan and Wicks 1990).

Different types of lone parent family

Lone parent families are sometimes seen and treated as an homogeneous group. At other times, they are divided into different sub-groups. Researchers and policy-makers often distinguish between different types of lone parent family according to their gender and marital status. A number of categorisations are possible but most begin by separating out lone fathers and widowed lone mothers from the rest. The remaining lone mothers are then quite often divided according to their marital or relationship history. Categorisations using marriage as the main factor distinguish between those who have separated or divorced from a husband and those who have never been married. Other categorisations take account of cohabitation and distinguish between those who have ever lived with a partner and those who have not. One of the main difficulties for all these systems of categorisation is that people's lives are very complex. Imagine a woman who got married and then divorced without having any children. She then has a child while single. Would she be counted as a divorced lone mother or a single lone mother? According to many official classifications she would be counted as a divorced lone mother even though the circumstances in which she became a lone mother have more in common with single, never-married lone mothers.

It is important to consider why we make distinctions between groups such as never-married lone mothers and widows and divorced lone mothers. One possible reason might be to split lone parents into 'deserving' and 'undeserving' types. Widows are seen as the most deserving group followed by women whose husbands have left them. There is also likely to be a fair degree of public sympathy for lone fathers as these men have to take on a parenting role that is not seen as 'naturally' theirs. The least deserving group are often thought to be wives who leave their husbands and women who have babies while single. This is because they appear to have been responsible for becoming a lone parent rather than being the victims of fate or unreliable partners. These groups are also most likely to be from working class backgrounds and be dependent on the state.

Distinctions based on marital status can therefore be used to divide lone parents into 'deserving'and 'undeserving' groups but these distinctions can also be useful in policy terms because policies towards lone parents may need to vary depending on the type of lone parent. As we shall see, single lone mothers are the most disadvantaged group. They come from poor backgrounds and they have poor future prospects. They may need particular social policies developed to meet their needs.

Marsh *et al.* (2001) offer the following typology from their 1999 survey of lone parents and low-income families (SOLIF):

1. Lone fathers.

2. Divorced mothers.

3. Mothers separated from a husband.

4. Mothers separated from a cohabiting partner.

5. Single lone mothers (women who have had no partner since the birth of their oldest dependent child).

6. Widowed mothers (bereaved either from husband or cohabiting partner).

Thus lone fathers (group 1) are treated as a whole and not divided further on the basis of current or previous marital status. This is because of their relatively small numbers. Widowed mothers (group 6) are also treated as a single group. The remaining lone parent families are then categorised on the basis of marital status. As argued above, there is a debate as to whether lone mothers who have previously been married (groups 2 and 3, according to Marsh *et al.* 2001) should be seen as distinctly different from those who have not (groups 4 and 5). An alternative approach is to make a distinction between those who have previously had a partner (groups 2, 3 and 4) and those who have not (5).

Using the typology from Marsh *et al.* (2001), lone parent families in 1999 fell into the following groups as shown in Figure 1.1.

Figure 1.1 shows that about half of all lone parent families in 1999 comprised women who had never been married (49 per cent). Over half of these had separated from a cohabiting partner (that is, 26 per cent of all lone parents), the rest (23 per cent) were women who had had a baby while living alone. Some of these may have cohabited in the past but not since the birth of their eldest child. About four lone parents in ten (42 per cent) were separated or divorced from a husband. As we shall see,

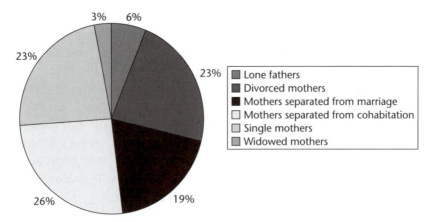

Figure 1.1 Lone parent families by gender and marital status in 1999.
Source: SOLIF 1999 (Marsh *et al.* 2001: Table 2.2)

mothers separated or divorced from a husband are quite similar to each other not least because the distinction between these two groups is mostly a matter of timing – most mothers separated from marriage will become divorced mothers eventually. We shall therefore refer to them as the ex-married lone mothers and this group is, in many ways, rather different from single mothers. Those separated from a cohabitation appear to form a distinct group on their own. On some indicators they have more in common with the single lone mothers and on some they seem to have more in common with the ex-married lone mothers.

This section of the book draws heavily on the SOLIF study as it provides the most up-to-date and comprehensive data on lone parents in Britain. It comprised a survey of 2,800 lone parents and was carried out in 1999 by the Policy Studies Institute for the Department of Social Security. It used Child Benefit records to sample a complete cross-section of lone parent families. Our analysis concentrates on these families but the SOLIF data also include information on low- and middle-income couple families in the bottom 40 per cent of the income distribution of families (see Appendix 1 for further information).

Ages of lone parents and their children

Many members of the media and the general public have a stereotypical image of a lone parent as being a young single woman with two or three children. The reality is quite different (see Figure 1.2). The average age for all lone parents in 1999 was 35. Single lone mothers in 1999 were the youngest of all lone parents and yet, on average, they were still

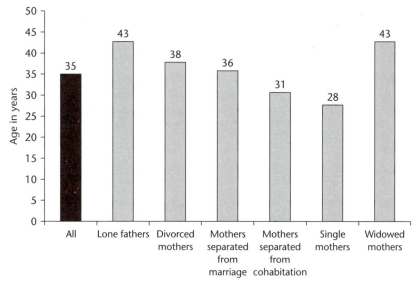

Figure 1.2 Average age of lone parents.
Source: SOLIF 1999 (Marsh *et al*. 2001: Table 2.6)

in their late 20s (Marsh *et al*. 2001). Lone mothers who had previously had a partner were more likely to be in their mid-30s and lone fathers and widowed lone mothers tended to be in their early 40s. Far from having numerous children, most lone parents only had one. And indeed single lone mothers were more likely than any other lone parent family type to have only one child (Figure 1.3).

There is great diversity among lone parent families in terms of whether or not they have pre-school-age children (see Figure 1.4). About half of lone mothers separated from cohabitation had children under 5 in 1999, rising to two-thirds among single lone mothers. Other lone parent families were much less likely to have children under the age of 5. This link between the route into lone parenthood and the age of the youngest child is quite easy to explain as single lone mothers become lone parents by having a baby. They do not remain lone parents forever and so it is not surprising that a high proportion have very young children. The age of the youngest child is a key factor in relation to employment status (see Chapter 6). Women with pre-school-age children (whether lone parents or not) are less likely to have paid jobs than those without. This is partly an issue of childcare and partly an issue of culture and identity – mothers with very young children are seen, and see themselves, as primarily responsible for the care of their children.

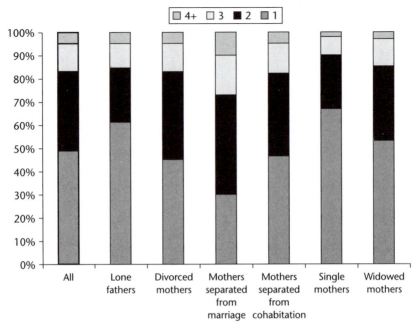

Figure 1.3 Average number of children.

Source: SOLIF 1999 (Marsh *et al.* 2001: Table 2.8)

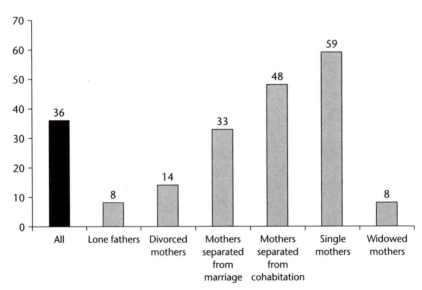

Figure 1.4 Lone parents with children of below school age.

Source: SOLIF 1999 (Marsh *et al.* 2001: Table 2.8)

Teenage lone mothers

We have just seen that lone parents are much older than is often imagined. This is partly because the media and government focus a great deal of attention on *teenage* lone mothers. More precisely, the government is concerned with teenage *pregnancy*. But it should be remembered that not all such pregnancies result in births and not all births are to single women. So the issue of teenage pregnancy does not equate directly to the issue of teenage lone mothers. Nevertheless it is worth reviewing both these issues. Britain has the highest rate of teenage births in Western Europe (Office of National Statistics 2001). Population Trends (1999) reveal that there were almost 90,000 conceptions to teenagers in England in 1997. Roughly three-fifths resulted in births (56,000), and 90 per cent of teenage births in 1997 were outside marriage (about 50,000).

According to our analysis of the *Family and Working Lives Survey* (FWLS) data, only 4 per cent of lone mothers in 1994–95 were aged between 16 and 19 years. While this might suggest that government attention on teenage lone parents might be out of proportion, other statistics suggest the opposite. For example, no fewer than 31 per cent of all lone mothers had their first child when a teenager, compared with 9 per cent of all mothers. Some of these births would have been within marriage and therefore would not, at that time, have represented teenage lone mother families. But people who marry young have a much greater risk of separation and divorce. Our analysis of FWLS also shows that just over half (56 per cent) of those who had been teenage mothers were, at the time, or went on to become, lone mothers, compared with 23 per cent of mothers who had children later than their teenage years. There is, therefore, good reason for any analysis of lone parenthood to look in detail at the circumstances surrounding early pregnancy and parenthood.

It is well known that teenage mothers tend to come from disadvantaged backgrounds. Our analysis of the *Family and Working Lives Survey* confirms this (see Table 1.1). Just 2 per cent of women with fathers in social class A (top professionals) and 5 per cent in social class B (senior managers and other professionals) became teenage mothers. This compares with 11 per cent overall, and as many as 23 per cent of women with unskilled fathers.

Data therefore suggest that very few current lone mothers are teenagers but a high proportion of teenage pregnancies lead to lone motherhood and a fairly high proportion of lone mothers were once teenage mothers. The Social Exclusion Unit (1999) draws on a range of evidence,

Table 1.1 Rates of teenage motherhood by social class of woman's father at age 16

Social class of father	Teenage mother (%)	Mother, at later age (%)	Not (yet) a mother (%)	Total (= 100 per cent)
A (senior professional)	2	65	33	103
B (professional)	5	59	37	609
C1 (clerical)	7	62	31	898
C2 (skilled manual)	12	65	24	1562
D (semi-skilled)	13	66	21	1117
E (unskilled)	23	52	25	191
Not working	15	45	40	57
Absent father or class unknown	16	60	24	540
All	**11**	**63**	**27**	**5077**

Source: own analysis of the *Family and Working Lives Survey* 1994–95

including that from Hobcraft and Kiernan (1999) to justify the attention paid to teenage pregnancy. They highlight the following factors:

- Higher infant mortality rates of babies and children born to teenage mothers.

- Higher rates of accidents among children of teenage mothers.

- Teenage mothers much more likely than other mothers to have no qualifications.

- Teenage mothers much more likely than other mothers to be on benefit or to have low incomes at the age of 33.

- Daughters of teenage mothers more likely than other girls to become teenage mothers themselves (though as a reason for interest in teenage parenthood it is rather circular).

The report gives three reasons why Britain has such a high rate of teenage pregnancy and lone motherhood. These are:

1. Low expectations: too many young people in Britain see no prospect of a job and fear that they will end up on benefit anyway – 'put simply, they see no reason not to get pregnant' (Social Exclusion Unit 1999: p. 7).

2. Ignorance: young people in Britain lack accurate knowledge about contraception, what to expect in relationships and what it means to get pregnant.

3.   Mixed messages: British culture as far as teenagers are concerned is contradictory – it may seem to them that 'sex is compulsory but contraception is illegal' (Social Exclusion Unit 1999: p. 7).

The report goes on to suggest various approaches to reduce 'the problem' of teenage pregnancy. Most of these approaches set out to tackle the problem of ignorance, and to some extent the problem of mixed messages. The Social Exclusion Unit (SEU) recommends various schemes that involve giving out information and advice but little is said about tackling the more fundamental issue of low expectations.

Teenage parenthood is therefore a major policy issue today but it is worth putting this into a broader historical and cultural context. In 1971, the teenage fertility rate was 50 per 100,000 compared with 28 per 100,000 in 1981 and 30 per 100,000 in 1999 (Office of National Statistics 2001). Thus teenage fertility has declined over time (but not to the same extent as it has declined in Europe). And the high rate of teenage fertility in the 1970s would mostly have been related to people marrying at very young ages. Some ethnic groups, such as Pakistanis and Bangladeshis, have very high rates of teenage motherhood (but very largely within marriage) (Berthoud 2001). Should this be considered a problem? Is it the age at which someone becomes a parent which is the issue or the age at which someone becomes a lone parent?

Ethnicity

The link between ethnicity and lone parenthood is an interesting and highly controversial one (see Song and Edwards 1996). The majority of lone parent families are white but some ethnic minorities are over-represented among lone parent families (such as Afro-Caribbean women) and others are under-represented (such as Asian women). In 1996, 6 per cent of the British population belonged to an ethnic minority group. In the 1999 SOLIF data however, a total of 9 per cent of lone parent families were from ethnic minority backgrounds. Five per cent of lone parent families were headed by a black lone parent, 2 per cent by an Asian lone parent and 2 per cent by a parent from another minority ethnic background.

The Labour Force Survey shows that just about two-thirds (66 per cent) of black Caribbean mothers were lone parents in 1995–97, compared with 21 per cent of white mothers (Holtermann et al. 1999). The majority (60 per cent) of black Caribbean lone mothers were single lone mothers, compared with only 6 per cent of Pakistani and Bangladeshi lone mothers. Lone motherhood in general, and single lone motherhood in particular, is very common within the black Caribbean community but it must be remembered that, according to the Labour Force Survey, black Caribbean women only constitute about 4 per cent of all lone mothers and only 6 per cent of all single lone mothers (Holtermann et al. 1999).

There is clearly a much higher rate of lone parenthood (and particularly single lone motherhood) among Caribbean women compared with white women. But it is difficult to make direct comparisons because these two groups of women are rather different in terms of a range of factors such as education, social class, age, age of children and so on. And there are important interactions between education and lone parenthood within the black as well as white communities. Berthoud (2000) has found that only one in ten Caribbean women with degree-level qualifications had become single lone mothers compared with almost half who had no qualifications. The same analysis applied to white women found only 2 per cent of those with degrees had become single lone mothers compared with 12 per cent of those with no qualifications.

The reason for high rates of lone parenthood among the Caribbean community must be understood within the context of differences in family patterns and culture between this community and the white and South Asian communities. The Caribbean community has very low rates of cohabitation and marriage compared with white men and women. In the early 1990s, only 39 per cent of Caribbean adults under 60 were married compared with 60 per cent of white adults (Berthoud 2000). By contrast, the South Asian community has a very high rate of marriage with three-quarters of Pakistani and Bangladeshi women married by the age of 25 (78 per cent and 71 per cent respectively). The same is true for two-thirds of Indian women (67 per cent) and only half of all white women (55 per cent). And separation and divorce are much less common in the South Asian community.

Culture, tradition and religion vary considerably between the white, Caribbean and South Asian communities. In West Indian life, 'visiting relationships' between fathers and their families have been a traditional feature. Matriarchal family structures have also been strong in this community and there is some evidence that more emphasis has traditionally been placed on individual choice and idealised marriage compared with the white community (Beishon et al. 1998). However, it is interesting to note that the behaviour said to derive from West Indian life is becoming more common in Britain. Second generation Caribbeans in Britain are more likely to live in what has been called a Caribbean/West Indian traditional lifestyle than the first generation. So perhaps it is more accurate to consider these living arrangements as part of 'British Caribbean' culture rather than simply Caribbean or West Indian culture. These characteristics of British Caribbean culture, according to some, have much in common with the 'modern individualist' nature of life in Britain today (Berthoud 2000). By contrast, South Asian culture generally has a more patriarchal nuclear family structure and heavily stigmatises divorce and illegitimacy. This resembles, to some extent, the 'traditional' Victorian values from which British society is departing.

There is evidence of a great deal of change in some family patterns within some ethnic groups. Berthoud (2001) has analysed teenage births to ethnic minority women and found that in the late 1970s/early 1980s, there were widespread differences between ethnic groups in terms of teenage births. Indian women had the lowest rates of teenage births (22 per thousand) followed closely by white women (27 per thousand). Caribbean women were somewhat higher (46 per thousand) with Pakistani women higher again (62 per thousand). Bangladeshi women had the very highest levels (83 per thousand). By the early/mid-1990s, these figures had changed considerably for some groups. For example, the rate of teenage birth had dropped dramatically for both Indian women (to 7 per thousand) and Bangladeshi women (to 53 per thousand). This meant that there was now very little difference between the teenage birth rates of Caribbean women and Bangladeshi women – though there are great differences in marriage patterns (as mentioned above).

Health, housing and hardship

Another characteristic of lone parent families that often goes unreported is their poor health (see Chapter 9). Three lone parents in ten had at least one long-standing health problem in 1999 (Marsh *et al.* 2001). Those out of work were more likely to have health problems than those in work. As well as having their own children to care for, 9 per cent of lone parents also cared for a sick or disabled relative or friend. The cause and effect relationship between lone parenthood and health is an interesting one. Do illness and impairment contribute to the creation of lone parent families (perhaps placing strains on relationships)? Or does lone parenthood itself somehow cause ill health and impairment (perhaps due to the strains of life as a lone parent)? It is likely that both mechanisms are at work.

The majority of the general public now own their own homes (or at least have a mortgage) but this is not the case for lone parents. Just over a quarter were home-owners (with or without a mortgage) and around two-thirds were tenants (most of these being social tenants) in 1999. Single lone mothers and women who had separated from a cohabiting partner were much more likely to be tenants than other types of lone parent. The issue of housing tenure touches on one stereotype of lone parents

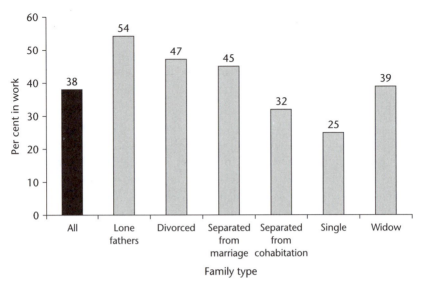

Figure 1.5 Percentage of different family types in paid work (16+ hours).
Source: SOLIF 1999 (Marsh *et al.* 2001: Table 2.21)

– that of women who deliberately become lone parents to get a faster route to council accommodation. It also confounds an alternative stereotype of lone parents, albeit now less common, of relatively comfortable women gaining a house at the expense of their partners who move out into poorer accommodation (see Chapter 9 for further discussion of these issues).

Another important aspect of lone parents is their poor financial status. This is partly dictated by their work status: the majority of lone parents (62 per cent) did not have paid work (or at least did not work 16 hours a week or more) in 1999. Most of those not in paid work were looking after their home or family but some lone parents (6 per cent) were doing a few hours paid work a week, some (5 per cent) were unemployed and seeking work, some classified themselves as sick or disabled (5 per cent) and a few (2 per cent) were in full-time education. Single lone mothers were least likely to work, followed by mothers separated from a cohabiting partner. Those most likely to work were lone fathers and lone mothers who had previously been married (see Figure 1.5). Of all groups, lone fathers were most likely to have high or moderate incomes. A gender dimension is relevant here in that lone fathers were among the most likely to work. But their rates of working fall short of fathers in two-parent families. There is also a strong link between work and having previously been married – though this may arise through the ex-marrieds tending to have older children on average, and for themselves to be older too.

One of the reasons why many lone parents are not in paid work is that they have low levels of education and qualifications (for example, compared with married mothers). In 1999, almost three lone parents in four (73 per cent) had left full-time education at or before the age of 16. Thirty-seven per cent had left without any formal qualifications. For 31 per cent their highest formal qualification included GCSEs graded A to C. The highest qualification for a further 7 per cent was A levels. And a further 6 per cent had degrees.

The result of low employment rates in Britain is poverty. Of all children living in a lone parent family in 1998/99, nearly four in five had incomes in the bottom 40 per cent of the distribution (Department of Social Security 2000). Similarly, over three-quarters of individuals in lone parent families were in the bottom 40 per cent of the income distribution. So the majority, the vast majority of children in lone parent families live in low-income families.

But what about poverty? Well there are lots of ways of measuring poverty but a standard way of doing it is to say that anyone living on an income which is below half the average income in the country is living in poverty. On this measure 62 per cent of children living in lone parent households were living in poverty in 1998/99 (Department of Social Security 2000). This adds up to 1.8 million children. The rate for children as a whole is one in three (34 per cent) which adds up to about 3.8 million children. This means that if you look at all poor children together, about half (48 per cent) lived in lone parent families in 1998/99.

Box 1.2   Lone parent families are poor families

- Nearly four in five children in lone parent families have incomes in the bottom 40 per cent of the distribution.
- 62 per cent of children living in lone parent households live in poverty (in households with below half average income after housing costs).
- The equivalent figure for all children is one in three (34 per cent).
- Nearly half of all poor children (1.8 million out of a total of 3.8 million) live in lone parent families.

Source: *Households Below Average Incomes* 1998/99 (Department of Social Security 2000)

Note: These figures are based on the measure taken after housing costs, and exclude the self-employed.

Social class

We have already looked at joblessness and poverty so we have touched on issues of social disadvantage but joblessness and poverty are not the same as social class. Now we turn specifically to social class and reveal the results of some new analysis of the Family and Working Lives Survey (FWLS) 1994/95 (see Appendix 1 for further details of this data source). Our analysis of FWLS begins by looking at the chances that a woman will have a baby before marrying or cohabiting with a partner. This is not the same as the definition of a 'single lone parent' in most official statistics as the official definition will include people who have separated from a cohabitation and then had a baby while living alone. Our 'single lone mothers' are therefore not only single at the point they have their babies but have never lived with a partner.

Using this approach we find that 7 per cent of women in the survey had, at some point in their lives, become a single lone mother. That is, they had given birth to a child prior to *any* marriage or cohabitation. But how does this vary by social class? There are a number of ways we could seek to answer this question. For example, we could look at the social class of the woman at the time she had the baby (or some time thereafter) or at the time she conceived the baby. But we are equally interested in the background from which the woman came. As suggested by the SEU's report on teenage pregnancy (Social Exclusion Unit 1999), young women often become lone parents due to low expectations and so it is their background that we wish to capture in our analysis of social class. We have therefore looked at the social class of the lone mother's father at the time she was 16. Figure 1.6 illustrates our findings. The chances of becoming a single lone mother were very low among women of professional fathers and increased as we move down the social class scale towards unskilled workers. A 16-year-old girl with an unskilled manual working father had six times the chance of becoming a single lone mother as a 16-year-old girl with a father in a professional occupation.

Social class has traditionally been measured by classifying the occupation of the (male) head of the household. With the growth of lone parenthood, however, not all households have a man in them. Our analysis of father's social class found that about one 16-year-old in ten either did not have a father in the household or had a father whose social grade could not be classified. Girls in this situation had a much higher than average chance of becoming a single lone mother – but no higher than girls with unemployed or unskilled fathers.

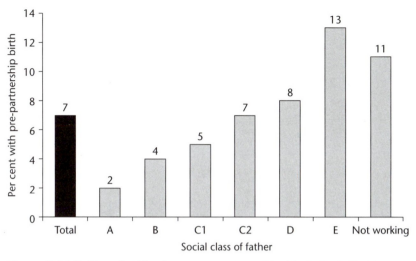

Figure 1.6 Likelihood of having a pre-partnership birth, by father's social class.

Source: Authors' own analysis of the *Family and Working Life Survey* 1994/95

The traditional focus on the male head of the household is open to criticism owing to the rise in women working and the apparent increase in equality between men and women generally. Thus we repeated our initial analysis but this time focused on the social class of *mothers* of 16-year-old girls. This shows us a similar picture as the analysis of fathers – the chances of becoming a single lone mother are much greater for girls with working class mothers than those with middle class mothers.

Another way of addressing this question is to focus on all those women in the survey who became single lone mothers (that is, single women who had babies without ever living with a partner) and analyse the social class background they came from (see Table 1.2). This shows us that only one in five single lone mothers came from a middle class background and most of these middle class girls had junior non-manual working fathers rather than fathers in the professions. In total, two-thirds of single lone mothers had working class fathers and a further 15 per cent either had no father at home at the age of 16 or his social grade could not be classified for some reason.

The other main route into lone parenthood is through the break-down of a marriage or cohabitation where there are children. In Table 1.2, the social profile of those women entering lone parenthood through this route looks closer to the profile of all women, but still with a slight tend-ency for this group to be more working class than average. Those who be-came single lone mothers, the group discussed above, have been taken out of this analysis. In other words, what is probably the most disadvantaged

Table 1.2 Social class background of women who became lone mothers

	Women who became single lone mothers (%)	Women becoming lone mothers after marriage or cohabitation (%)	All women (%)
Social class of father when woman was 16			
A (senior professional)	1	2	2
B (professional)	7	10	13
C1 (clerical)	13	16	18
C2 (skilled manual)	29	29	31
D (semi-skilled)	27	25	21
E (unskilled)	7	5	4
Not working	2	1	1
Not present in family/not known	15	12	10
Summary			
Middle class (ABC1)	21	28	33
Working class (C2DE)	65	60	57
Absent or unknown	15	12	10

Source: Authors' own analysis of *Family and Working Lives Survey* 1994/95

group has been removed, and still there is some effect of class background on rates of separation. Had they been included, the effects of parental background on rates of separation would, probably, have been still larger. Of course, the event of separating from a partner will generally be many years removed from social status at the age of 16 and so perhaps this is a less valid way of measuring social class for this group but it is interesting to make the comparison and the analysis is still useful.

Further analysis of the FWLS showed that one in five couples with children separated to form a lone mother unit. The *rate* of relationship breakdown to form a lone parent family was much higher than average, at 31 per cent, for those from an unskilled working class background, and slightly lower (at 17 per cent) for those from social classes B (senior managers and professionals) and C1 (other non-manual workers).

1.2 The dynamics of lone parenthood

Children rarely experience lone parenthood for the whole of their childhoods. Similarly, lone parenthood does not last forever for the parent. People may cease being lone parents when their children become older (and hence are no longer counted as dependent), or through living with a partner – the route through which most spells of lone motherhood end.

Table 1.3 The average (median) duration (in months) of lone motherhood by marital status

	WES 1980: life history data (Ermisch 1991)	SCELI life history data 1986 (Rowlingson and McKay 1998)	BHPS life history data 1992: from transition rates (Böheim and Ermisch 1998)	BHPS panel data 1991–95: from transition rates (Böheim and Ermisch 1998)	Family and Working Lives Survey 1994/95 (own analysis)
Status of lone mother					
Single	35	38	20	55	55
Divorced	} 59	56	} 64	} 52	56
Separated		102			82
Widowed	–	–	–	–	126
Overall duration	–	–	–	–	70

Note: The two BHPS estimates are derived from transition rates. The other estimates are based on life-table estimation.

According to Rowlingson and McKay (1998), half of all lone parents leave lone parenthood within six years of becoming a lone parent. Single lone mothers have shorter spells of lone parenthood than other types of lone parent – about half of all single lone mothers marry within three years of giving birth to the child that made them a lone mother.

However, there is evidence that the duration of lone motherhood, for those counted as 'single', has increased substantially compared with previous (dated) evidence. Table 1.3 compares the results from a number of studies based on data from surveys covering 1980 to 1995. The median duration as a single lone mother (the time within which half would be expected to change status) has risen from around three years, to closer to five years using the most recent evidence. The estimated duration of lone motherhood for divorced women appears to have hardly changed.

Drawing on a cross-section of lone parents in 1991, one study found that eight out of ten lone parents were still alone in 1995 (Ford et al. 1998). A few of these had joined but then left a partner in the intervening years. Most of the remainder were with new partners but some had got back together with ex-partners, usually (ex-)husbands. Fourteen per cent of 1991 lone parents no longer had dependent children in 1995 and so were no longer lone parents. In most cases, the children had simply grown up but remained in the same household. One in five had had new babies or were expecting one soon. Half of these new children were (about to be) born within a partnership but half were not. Logistic regression analysis suggested that younger women, or those with older children, were most likely to leave lone parenthood. Thus never-married lone parents had a high rate of (re-)partnering because of their age.

Another study found that housing tenure was important in relation to (re-)partnering as lone parents who were owner-occupiers remained lone parents for shorter spells than those who rented their homes (Rowlingson and McKay 1998). It is not clear why this link exists – perhaps owner-occupying women are more attractive to potential partners.

The analysis so far has looked at the types of people who leave, or remain in, lone parenthood. It takes a fairly structural approach to the question and has little to say about the decisions people make in their lives and the reasons they might choose to stay as lone parents or move in with a partner. Other analysis investigates the role of human agency and choice in this field. It asks the question: how do people feel about being lone parents? And do they want to remain in this position? Bradshaw and Millar (1991) asked their sample for the best and worst things about being a lone parent. Among the advantages cited were independence and freedom. These were particularly important to people who had previously been part of a couple. Having peace of mind and a peaceful household was also import-ant to many. About one lone parent in ten felt that one of the best things was the ability to manage one's own money and once again it was lone parents who had previously lived with a partner who particularly appre-ciated this aspect of lone parenthood. However, one of the greatest dis-advantages was lack of money – nearly half of all lone parents mentioned financial difficulties as one of the worst aspects of lone parenthood. A more widespread disadvantage, however, was loneliness (see Table 1.4).

Qualitative research has also explored why people leave or remain in lone parenthood (Rowlingson and McKay 1998). The findings echo those from the quantitative research just mentioned. A number of lone mothers explained why they were happy to remain as lone parents:

Table 1.4 Best things and worst things about being a lone parent

Best things	Percentage	Worst things	Percentage
Own boss/independence	60	Loneliness	48
Freedom to do what you want	31	Financial difficulties	45
Own decisions for children	21	Coping with children	30
Peace of mind	15	No one to discuss problems with	15
Household peaceful	13	Lack of adult conversation	12
Cope better with money	12	Miss being in a couple	12
More time for children/self	10	Socially hard	12

Source: from Bradshaw and Millar (1991)

'I just don't want any man telling me what to do any more and taking over my life because it's nice to feel free and able to do what you like.'   (p. 166)

'That house has always been my space, and then to have someone come into that space, like day in and day out – it's scary!'   (p. 167)

'It's nice that I'm solely responsible for bringing the boys up and what I say goes.'   (p. 163)

'I'm not as badly off as I thought I was because I can manage my finances and it's only me that looks after the finances.'   (p. 160)

But some lone mothers were not so happy with their lives and would have been more interested in finding a partner:

'It would be nice just to like have someone what is like close to you, with you, sort of thing, just to like talk to.'   (p. 164)

'You've got all the worry of – well everything. You've got your bill worries – all that's your own. You've got your children – all that's your own. Every worry that you ever get, which everybody gets, you have to deal with it yourself.'   (p. 165)

'Sometimes it's been hard . . . having to sit and count your money out at the end of the week and then [my daughter] needs something like a pair of shoes and things like that and you think to yourself, 'God, where am I going to get the money from for a pair of shoes?'

(p. 158)

'I need a man around for my son's sake . . . now is the stage that [my son] needs a man in his life. But I don't.'   (p. 172)

'I don't want to grow old and be on my own.'   (p. 171)

Some people want to remain lone parents because they feel that the advantages outweigh the disadvantages. Others make a different calculation and so are keen to leave lone parenthood. But even those who are keen to leave lone parenthood still have to find a partner. And many are only prepared to accept a partner if that person meets their specific requirements.

Some women (and their children) move in and out of lone parenthood a number of times. For example, they might have a baby while single but then get married a few years later. A few years after getting married they might have another child and a few years after this they might separate and divorce from their husband and so on. It is very difficult to quantify how common such movements in and out of lone parenthood are.

1.3 A profile of non-resident parents

We know a great deal about lone parents and their children as there have been numerous quantitative and qualitative studies that have involved them. Non-resident parents, however, are a much less-researched group. This is partly because, unlike lone parent families, they have not been considered to be a social problem until recently. Their emergence as a social problem coincides with the debate about child support payments and, in particular, the fact that they pay relatively little in maintenance. Another reason for the lack of research is that they are a difficult group to locate for research purposes. Lone parents have formed interest groups or pressure groups (like the National Council for One Parent Families and Gingerbread) for decades now and so they have been easy to find for small-scale studies. For larger, representative surveys, lone parents can be found by writing to people who receive Child Benefit and selecting the lone parents. Non-resident parents are a much more difficult group to find: until the 1980s there were very few support groups for them and they are not, as a whole, dependent on particular public services.

The main way of solving this problem is to interview a representative sample of the general public and then ask all adults whether or not they are the parent of a child that lives in a household other than their own. Those who say they are may then be interviewed further. But will all non-resident fathers tell a survey interviewer that they have a child in another household? There is some stigma attached to being a non-resident parent, especially if there is little contact with the child. And if the non-resident parent is not paying any maintenance, there may be fears of being reported to the Child Support Agency. Some men may not even know that they have fathered a child in another household. It is likely that surveys employing this method will under-represent younger, poorer, never-married nonresident fathers. The survey method therefore poses problems but it has provided among the best information we have about non-resident parents.

A group at the University of York used just such a method to identify a sample of non-resident fathers. Bearing in mind all the reservations mentioned above, Bradshaw et al.'s (1999) study of non-resident fathers gives a profile of this group, shown in Table 1.5. This table also gives comparative information on a sample of all fathers from the Family Resources Survey in 1994/95. The survey shows that non-resident fathers are a little younger than all fathers: they are more likely to be under 35 and less likely to be 35 or over (as compared with all fathers). More than a third of non-resident fathers live on their own (36 per cent), 16 per cent live with a

Table 1.5 Characteristics of non-resident fathers in 1996 survey by Bradshaw *et al.* (1999) and all fathers in FRS 1994/95

	Non-resident fathers in 1996 (%)	All fathers (FRS 1994/95) (%)
Age		
Under 25	5	3
25–30	14	14
31–34	25	17
35–40	23	27
41–49	28	30
50+	5	10
Household composition		
Living alone	36	
Living with a partner only	16	
Living with partner and children	26	
Living with children only	4	
Living with relatives	9	
Other	9	
Social class		
Professional/intermediate	19	27
Other non-manual	17	18
Skilled manual	30	38
Semi-skilled manual	19	14
Unskilled manual	15	5
Qualifications		
No qualifications	32	

Source: Bradshaw *et al.* (1999)

partner but no children and more than a quarter (26 per cent) live with a new partner and children. A few non-resident fathers (4 per cent) are also lone parents themselves. In terms of their socio-economic or class profile, non-resident fathers are much more working class than the average father: they are three times as likely to be unskilled manual workers. This position is reflected in the fact that almost one-third of non-resident fathers have no qualifications.

Another source of large-scale data on non-resident parents is the Child Support Agency (CSA). This organisation has carried out satisfaction surveys of the parents they have been in contact with and these surveys provide profiles of non-resident parents. This group of non-resident parents is unlikely to be representative of all non-resident parents as some will not have had contact with the CSA (for example, if their former partner/lover is not on Income Support). And some will have evaded the CSA (for example if their former partner/lover has not told the CSA who they are

Table 1.6 Characteristics of non-resident parents in contact with the CSA in 1994

	Per cent
Age	
16–24	7
25–34	41
35–44	38
45–54	13
55+	1
Current marital status	
Single	20
Separated	10
Divorced	26
Married	25
Living with new partner	17
Previous relationship	
Husband/wife	66
Cohabiting partner	21
Boyfriend/girlfriend	11
Casual relationship	2
No relationship/other	2
Socio-economic group	
AB (Professionals, managers)	6
C1 (Non-manual workers)	19
C2 (Skilled manual workers)	22
DE (Un/semi-skilled/jobless)	54
Work status	
Employed	64
Looking for work	18
Economically inactive	17
Qualifications	
No qualifications	35

Source: Speed and Kent (1996)

or they have been difficult to track down). Despite its limitations, it is nevertheless interesting to look at the CSA's profile of non-resident parents (see Table 1.6, Speed and Kent 1996). Unlike the survey by Bradshaw *et al.* (1999), the CSA profile includes non-resident *mothers* as well as fathers but non-resident parents were overwhelmingly male (96 per cent). Almost eight in ten were between 25 and 44, with an average age of 36. Their previous relationship history shows that while two-thirds had been married, one in five had been cohabiting and one in ten had simply been boyfriends or girlfriends. Only a handful had been in very casual relationships.

Over half of all non-resident parents known to the CSA were in social class DE (unskilled or semi-skilled manual work or unemployed/inactive). A further one in five were skilled manual workers. Three-quarters were therefore working class. Following on from this, almost two-thirds were in paid work but almost one in five were unemployed and a further 17 per cent were economically inactive. One in five were on Income Support. Just over a third had no qualifications at all.

It is interesting to compare this profile with that provided by Bradshaw *et al.* (1999) though it is difficult to compare directly as the information has been collected and presented in slightly different ways. The CSA profile broadly reflects that shown in Bradshaw *et al.* (1999) but the CSA group appears to be more working class. Only 6 per cent of the CSA group were in professional or managerial occupations compared with 19 per cent of non-resident fathers in the Bradshaw *et al.* (1999) study and 27 per cent of all fathers in Britain. This probably reflects the particular client base of the CSA but it might also be due to the method used by Bradshaw *et al.* – middle class non-resident fathers were probably more likely to admit their status and take part in the study.

1.4 International comparisons

So far this book has concentrated on lone parent families in Britain today. We now take a look at some other countries to see that recent trends in Britain are by no means unique. First, we look at empirical findings from studies of different countries and then we look at more theoretical models of variations between countries.

Empirical findings

The growth of lone parenthood is not unique to Britain – the trend is common to many advanced industrial countries, as are trends towards increasing cohabitation, increasing divorce and increasing numbers of births outside marriage. Nevertheless in 1990, Britain had one of the highest rates of lone motherhood in Europe along with Sweden, Norway and Denmark (Whiteford and Bradshaw 1994). The European countries with some of the lowest levels include Greece, Ireland, Italy, Portugal and Spain. This division suggests some combination of North/South, rich/poor, Protestant/Catholic factors at work. Countries that are generally rich Protestant North European countries have much higher rates of lone parenthood than those that are mainly poor Southern Catholic countries (see Figure 1.7), though Britain cuts across this division as it is a relatively poor country but is

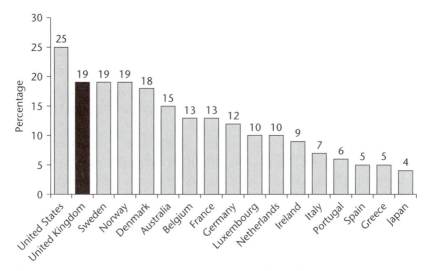

Figure 1.7 Lone parents as a proportion of all families with children in 1990.

Source: Whiteford and Bradshaw (1994)

Northern and Protestant. Culture and religion therefore seem important factors when seeking to explain variations in rates of lone parenthood. If we look outside Europe but remain within the developed world, Japan has a very low rate of lone parenthood, Australia has a slightly lower rate than Britain and the USA has by far the highest rate.

The percentage of births outside marriage also varies substantially by country. This figure cannot be taken as a direct indicator of lone parenthood as these births could be to cohabiting parents, and clearly usually are, but there does appear to be some correlation as the highest rates of births outside marriage are in Denmark, Norway and Sweden. The lowest rates are in Greece and Italy. The UK and the USA fall somewhere in between these two extremes. Divorce rates are also associated with lone parenthood. The highest rates are in Denmark, UK and Sweden with the lowest rates in Greece, Ireland, Italy, Portugal and Spain. The United States has by far the highest rate.

Another interesting point of comparison is the family marital status of lone parents within each country. For example, the proportion of lone parents who are never married varies dramatically from more than half in Norway and Sweden to about a third in the USA and UK. Never-married lone parents are virtually non-existent in Greece, Portugal and Japan (Table 1.7).

There is also a great deal of variation in the employment patterns of lone parents across different countries (see Figure 1.8). The Netherlands, UK and Ireland have the lowest rates of full-time paid work for lone parents: fewer than one in five lone parents in these countries have a paid

Table 1.7 Summary of demographic differences between countries

	Highest	Lowest
Rates of lone parenthood	UK, Sweden, Norway, Demark, USA, Australia	Greece, Ireland, Italy, Portugal, Spain, Japan
Percentage of births outside marriage	Denmark, Norway, Sweden	Greece, Italy, Japan
Divorce rates	UK, Sweden, Denmark, USA	Greece, Ireland, Italy, Portugal, Spain, Japan
Percentage of lone parents who are never-married	Norway and Sweden (then USA and UK)	Greece, Portugal and Japan

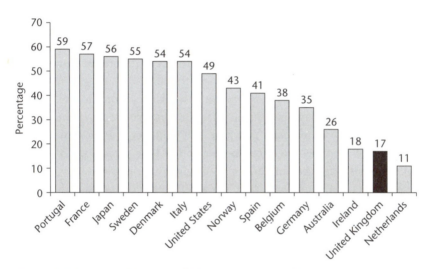

Figure 1.8 Lone mothers in full-time employment by country.
Source: Whiteford and Bradshaw (1994)

job. The highest rates are found in Portugal, France, Japan, Italy, Sweden and Denmark – where over half of all lone parents work full-time. The reasons for these variations will be discussed below. Overall, however, lone mothers in all countries apart from the UK are either more likely to be working full-time than all mothers or the level of full-time employment is about the same. And generally, lone mothers are less likely to work part-time than all mothers.

Cross-national studies have been used to throw light on the relationship between social security benefits and lone parenthood. It is common for those on the political right to argue that lone parenthood has risen because women have access to relatively high rates of benefit. Whiteford and Bradshaw (1994) found some evidence that appeared to support this view. For example, Greece and Portugal had low levels of social security support for lone parents and also low levels of lone parenthood. At the other end of the spectrum, Norway, Denmark and Australia had higher levels of both social assistance and lone parenthood. But Whiteford and Bradshaw warn against moving too swiftly from this association to drawing conclusions about causation. It is possible that the high rates of benefit in some countries were the *result* of a growth in lone parenthood (due to a growing lobby group and increasing recognition of the need for higher benefits) rather than the *cause* of the growth. Also, the USA provides an important exception to any correlation between levels of lone parenthood and levels of benefit. As we have seen, the USA has the highest level of lone parenthood in the Western world but its level of social assistance is among the lowest (lower even than that available in Ireland and Spain). Bradshaw and Whiteford (1994) therefore concluded that there was only a weak association between high rates of benefits for lone parents and high rates of lone parenthood.

Social security policy may have only weak effects on the *rate* of lone parenthood but it may nevertheless affect the *employment participation* rates of lone parents. Here again, however, the evidence is inconclusive. For example, Sweden has the largest proportion of lone parents in paid work but the benefit replacement rate is also the highest. This means that Swedish lone parents, compared with lone parents in other countries, will not be much better off financially in work than on benefit. We might therefore expect them to have low employment rates but they do not. This therefore contradicts a narrow rational economic model of behaviour that assumes people weigh up the financial costs and benefits of a particular course of action and then act accordingly. France and Germany on the other hand have relatively high proportions of lone parents in work along with relatively low benefit replacement rates (thus supporting the rational economic model). Denmark and France have similar proportions of lone parents in the labour force but Denmark is relatively generous to lone parents on benefit whereas France is relatively mean.

Whiteford and Bradshaw (1994) put forward a range of possible explanatory factors relating to Denmark's high rate of employment alongside its generous benefit levels:

- high level of publicly funded childcare;
- provision of advanced maintenance;
- high level of earnings equality between men and women;
- high lone parent premiums;
- high real average wage levels.

An interesting aspect of the French system of social security is that it is much more generous to lone parents with young children whether or not they are in paid work. Those with older children are given much less help. This could have the effect of encouraging new lone parents to carry on working and other lone parents to take up or stay in paid work.

The overall conclusion from Whiteford and Bradshaw's work (1994: p. 86) is that 'the aspirations of lone parents to work are related to the general labour force position of women.' Thus there are links between all mothers, lone mothers and employment rates. This supports a gendered approach to lone parenthood and also questions the appropriateness of singling out lone mothers as a group. If the experience of lone mothers is just an extreme version of that for all mothers, then perhaps policies should be aimed at improving the opportunities of all mothers rather than just focusing on lone mothers in particular. Or perhaps policies could be aimed at those (both women and men) with poorer educational and employment prospects.

Other research (Millar and Rowlingson 2001) has analysed how different countries have approached the issue of lone parents and employment. Most advanced industrial countries are increasingly encouraging (if not compelling) lone parents to enter the labour market. But the ways in which they do this vary. Some, such as the USA, aim to achieve this largely by restricting access to benefits. Others, such as the UK, attempt to 'make work pay' principally through in-work benefits. And others, such as Norway, provide cheap childcare. These policies have been most successful where they fit with lone parents' own aspirations about employment. In the Netherlands, for example, a new policy to encourage lone parents into employment has largely failed because neither lone parents themselves nor their employment advisers nor society more generally, really felt it appropriate to push lone parents (back) into the labour market (Knijn and van Wel 2001). Similarly, Duncan and Edwards (1999) highlight the role of social context in determining whether or not lone mothers take paid work. Social and cultural norms about mothers as carers or workers have a major impact on employment patterns.

Welfare regimes

Some researchers have tried to categorise countries into groups in terms of how women and lone parents fare in these different countries, especially in relation to employment and social policies. This general approach of categorising 'welfare regimes' is most heavily associated with Esping-Andersen (1990) who categorised welfare regimes in terms of the policy logics that revolved around a paid worker's dependence, or independence from, the labour market. A number of feminist researchers (Lewis 1992, Sainsbury 1996) have criticised this approach for focusing too heavily on male workers and thus ignoring the role of women in both paid and unpaid work. Lewis (1992) has proposed an alternative typology around the concept of breadwinning. This typology places countries into one of three categories: strong breadwinner regimes; modified breadwinner regimes; and weak breadwinner regimes.

At its extreme, the male breadwinner model involves the exclusion of women from the labour market. Women would be expected to do all unpaid caring work and they would be dependent on men for access to all income including social security payments. Lone parents would cause a problem in such a society as they have no breadwinner but do have children to support. Lewis with Hobson (1997) argue that the male breadwinner model is generally breaking down but that some countries do still have strong male breadwinner regimes such as the UK, USA, Germany, the Netherlands and Ireland. There is variation, however, even within this group in terms of the labour market participation of lone parents. Lewis with Hobson (1997) classify Sweden as a weak or dual breadwinner model – women, including lone parents, are expected to take on paid work while men are expected to take on unpaid work in the home. There is good childcare provision and employment of women is high. But there is also a relatively generous benefit system so that even when some people are out of work, levels of poverty are low.

The difficulties of classifying countries are evident when Lewis with Hobson (1997) invent a separate category to cover Italy – the 'intergenerational model'. This model encompasses countries where there is a great deal of importance placed on family support. In Italy, most lone parents are widows and they receive relatively generous state benefits. But there is little state support for other types of lone parent who must turn to their extended family for financial support and childcare. The role of the extended family means that lone parents in Italy have relatively high rates of employment.

Another way of classifying countries is in terms of whether they focus on lone parents as mothers (the 'caregiving' model) or workers (the 'parent/worker' model) (see Duncan and Edwards 1997). The Netherlands is a prime example of the former where sufficient support is given to lone parents to remain in the home to look after their children. The state therefore provides support for women as mothers. Lone parents are able to establish autonomous households without suffering poverty and deprivation and they can do so without having to engage with the labour market. Sweden, however, is an example of the parent/worker model. Lone parents here are also able to establish autonomous households without suffering poverty and deprivation but here they tend to do so through engaging with the labour market. The state provides support in terms of childcare, wages are relatively generous and there are reasonable benefit payments to those out of work.

The capacity for lone parents to establish autonomous households without suffering poverty and deprivation might be seen as a benchmark with which to measure gender (and class) equality in different countries (Orloff 1993). We have seen that there are different ways of doing this – we can support lone parents to stay at home and care for their children (by having generous benefits) or we can support lone parents to take up paid work (by having affordable childcare and keeping wage rates high). Perhaps there is also a middle way in terms of supporting lone parents to combine roles by means of packaging their income – some income from part-time work, some from benefits, some from maintenance. This is perhaps the approach taken in the UK, where in-work benefits such as Working Families Tax Credit (formerly Family Credit) enable lone parents to put together such a package. But in the UK, wage and benefit levels have been too low to avoid poverty for all but a minority of lone parents.

As argued above, many countries, including the UK, are moving further and further towards an emphasis on paid work rather than care as the route to autonomy for lone parents. But paid work is no guarantee against poverty, as is evident in Japan and the USA. The success of some countries, such as Sweden, in combining high employment rates with low poverty rates, is due to a number of factors. These factors are summarised by Duncan and Edwards (1997) echoing Whiteford and Bradshaw (1994):

- Lone parents are working full-time rather than part-time.
- Childcare provision is paid for by the state.
- There are long parental leave schemes.
- There is paid leave to be with sick children.
- There are strong social transfers (benefit payments) for those out of work.
- There is a state advanced maintenance scheme.

We cannot therefore simply move lone parents into paid work and expect poverty to be eradicated. Other policies, such as those relating to childcare and employment rights also need to be put in place.

1.5 Summary

Lone parent families are a mainstream family type – about three million children currently live in a lone parent family and about half of all children will experience life in a lone parent family at some point in their childhood.

About half of all lone parents are mothers who have never been married but over half of these had separated from a cohabiting partner. Thus the growth in never-married lone motherhood is partly related to the growth of cohabitation.

The average age of all lone parents in 1999 was 35. Single lone mothers were the youngest type of lone mother but they were, on average, in their late 20s. Fewer than 1 lone parent in 20 is a teenager.

Nine lone parents in ten are white but some ethnic minorities are over-represented in lone parent families (such as Afro-Caribbean women) and some are under-represented (such as Asian women). More than half of black families with children are lone parent families compared with about a quarter of white families.

Lone parent families are poor families. About two-thirds of children living in lone parent families are poor. This is about twice the rate for all children. Half of all poor children (1.8 million out of 3.8 million) live in lone parent families. This is partly because poverty causes lone parenthood and partly because lone parenthood causes (further) poverty.

Lone parenthood is not, usually, for life. Children rarely experience lone parenthood for the whole of their childhoods. About half of all lone mothers (re-)partner within about 6 years and rates of (re-)partnering are higher for single lone mothers.

Britain has a high rate of lone parenthood, a high rate of lone parent poverty and a low rate of lone parent employment. Some other countries have similarly high rates of lone parenthood but without the corresponding problem of poverty. The Netherlands, for example, provides sufficient support for lone parents to remain in the home to look after their children without suffering poverty. Employment rates are therefore relatively low but poverty is not high. Sweden also provides relatively generous benefit payments to lone parents not in employment but it also encourages lone parents to get paid jobs. Wages are relatively high and the state provides generous child care help so that women in paid work avoid poverty. These examples show that lone parenthood need not be synonymous with poverty. It is possible for lone parents to remain at home with their children and avoid poverty (as in the Dutch model) or to engage with the labour market and avoid poverty (as in the Swedish model). However, one of the explanations for the success of these countries is their overall level of class and gender equality. Greater equality is a fundamental prerequisite to reducing lone parent poverty.

chapter 2

The fall and rise of lone parenthood

Lone parenthood has become an important issue following the dramatic rise in the number of lone parent families over the last 30 years or so. Chapter 1 described the patterns of lone parenthood in Britain today. This chapter takes a broad historical perspective on lone parenthood and assesses the nature of the trends in lone parenthood since early modern times. This shows us that lone parenthood has been relatively common throughout the last few centuries. It only appears to be a new phenomenon because of the unusual predominance of the nuclear family in the 1950s. One aspect of lone parenthood is, however, fairly unique historically: the number of single women having babies without a partner.

2.1 The historical context

Over the second half of the twentieth century, some commentators warned of the impending 'death of the family' which they saw reflected in the growth of divorce, lone parenthood, illegitimacy, cohabitation and childlessness. Morgan argued that: 'Since the 1970s, a climate of hostility to the family has provided the general context in which its legal and economic foundations have been easily undermined.' (1995: p. 1.) Like many of those who fear the 'death of the family', Morgan takes a selective view of changes in family patterns. She compares current family patterns with the early 1950s, a time when family life seemed comparatively stable, based on a male breadwinner married to a female housewife. She then takes a further step by identifying this *particular* family type with *the family* in general. Thus the relative demise of this historically and culturally specific family type signals the death of the family. However, if we take a broader view of history, we can see that there has been great diversity in family patterns in past centuries. Lone parenthood was relatively uncommon in the first half of the twentieth century but it has not always been so uncommon.

Before 1753: informal 'marriage' and 'self-divorce'

Snell and Millar (1987) estimate that at the end of the eighteenth century and the beginning of the nineteenth, 19 per cent of all families with children were lone parent families, a figure not too far off today's levels. Furthermore, 30 per cent of all families receiving parish relief under the old Poor Law (that is, prior to 1834) were lone parent families.

Lone parenthood in the past was often caused by widowhood. Data suggest that the mean duration of a marriage (before the death of a partner) was 20 years (Houlbrooke 1984). Until the 1800s, people commonly died in their middle years rather than reaching old age. This means that during the late sixteenth and early seventeenth centuries about one-fifth of all householders were widowed. Most of these people were women (as women lived slightly longer, and married men who were slightly older). And most had children and so were lone parents (although not all children were dependent) when widowed. Poor women faced a bleak life as widows and mothers. Remarriage was therefore often essential. Custom dictated that bereaved spouses should mourn their loved ones for at least a year but economic necessity often cut short this period of mourning. Houlbrooke (1984), using a sample of parish registers, has found that 37 per cent of all women who had remarried, had done so within a year of losing their husband. For men, the percentage was 48. The mean period between bereavement and remarriage for women was about three years and, for men, two years.

Lone parent families could also be created through couples separating. Married couples who wished to separate could not necessarily be granted an annulment. So different forms of 'self-divorce' became practised. For example, if a husband failed to maintain a wife financially, she could return his ring and thus informally divorce him. Having said this, most self-divorce was more formal and not usually entered into lightly. The consent of both parties made such practices more straightforward but good cause was needed and witnesses were required to accept these reasons. In many communities, a fair degree of gender equality was operated in relation to self-divorce. Other practices, such as 'wife sales', were also a means to end an unhappy relationship. While these may not seem particularly egalitarian from a gender perspective, they were usually conducted only with the consent of both parties. It was a rite that allowed a woman to leave her husband for a new man, of her choice, while her ex-husband was then also free to marry again if he so chose. Macfarlane (1986) argues that a tiny group at the top of the socio-economic system were able to gain divorce by Act of Parliament, while those at the bottom could use self-divorce or wife-sale, but the rest were stuck. They could separate but there was no prospect of remarriage.

According to Houlbrooke (1984) a survey carried out in Norwich in 1570 found that 8.5 per cent of poor married women had been 'abandoned' by their husbands. Abbott (1993) argues that when times were hard in the sixteenth and seventeenth centuries poor men would leave their families to find work. The poorer the migrant, the further he would travel, increasing the likelihood of permanent separation. At a time when illiteracy was common and sending letters far too expensive, families soon lost touch with each other.

Lone parent families in pre-industrial Britain were not only created by widowhood and separation from husbands, cohabitation was also a widespread form of family life. Gillis (1985: p. 4) argues that 'working people had repeatedly experimented with forms of family life based exclusively on the conjugal bond, only to reject these in favour of arrangements more broadly constructed.' Thus Gillis implies that marriage is the experiment rather than the universal norm. Up to the twelfth century, there had been no legal marriage in England and Wales, only ritual and custom. Until 1753, a variety of 'self-marriage' rites existed alongside the Church of England ceremony. Stone (1990) identifies 'contract marriages' and 'clandestine marriages', both of which were recognised in the law of the land, if both falling short of the fully sanctioned religious marriage ceremony. Gillis (1985) describes a number of unofficial ceremonies, including the practice of jumping over a broom to seal marriage vows.

Common-law marriage was therefore relatively widespread. Hibbert (1987) suggests that there were many local variations but the main ingredient for binding two people together included having witnesses present when the couple verbally promised 'to take thee to my wife/husband'. It was also common practice for the man to kiss the woman at this time and give her a present (usually a ring). Clergymen were not necessarily involved in these marriages but even the presence of a clergyman did not necessarily signify a very formal marriage. In London, 'Fleet marriages' were notorious. These weddings were presided over by clergymen debtors in Fleet prison and they would marry virtually anyone in return for money. The 'ceremonies' took place in the prison chapel and even in surrounding taverns and houses. They were not illegal until the mid-eighteenth century.

The couple could have an official document if they wished and it might even be backdated to legitimise any children born before the wedding. 'Self-divorce' from such informal marriage was probably much easier than from a more formal marriage.

In 1753, Hardwicke's Marriage Act introduced marriage in secular law and thereby abolished self-marriage. The Act declared that only church marriages, conducted according to particular rules including the signing of the parish register, could be considered a binding marriage. A verbal promise was no longer enough. But informal practices continued unofficially until the end of the nineteenth century. The rise in cohabitation in the last few decades of the twentieth century might therefore be seen as a return to the tradition of finding temporary alternatives to official marriage ceremonies. Then, as now, cohabitation was often a precursor to marriage rather than an alternative.

Until the end of the nineteenth century, it was not uncommon for children to be born to women who were not officially married. These women may not have been lone parents – some would have been living with the father – but if the relationship did not last, these women would be left holding the baby. Gillis (1985: p. 127) notes that 'Women were becoming mothers before they became wives. Some were giving birth to several children and never marrying at all.' In these cases, women were not just having children in anticipation of marriage but without prospect of marriage. This, argues Gillis (1985: p. 127), was a new phenomenon in the eighteenth century and was due to two distinct sets of circumstances. The first was the economic structures of the time: 'levels of unwed motherhood were extremely high in . . . places where employment for women at or near home was most abundant.' The second was the support which the extended family and wider kinship networks gave to lone mothers and their children. Thus Gillis argues (1985: p. 128) that 'the ability and willingness of women to have children outside of wedlock was a product of familial and communal cohesion rather than breakdown.'

While Gillis implies that cohabitation was common, reliable historical statistics on this subject are non-existent and Stone (1990) disputes the extent of informal cohabiting unions prior to industrialisation. He argues that while these may have been common in Wales and remote parts of England, there is little evidence of such practices in more prosperous areas. And where property was involved, self-marriage was rare. However, Stone (1990: p. 65) himself quotes data relating to illegitimacy that show a phenomenal rise from 6 per cent of all first births in 1690 to 20 per cent in 1790. Many of these births, he argues, would then have prompted an official marriage but, nevertheless, illegitimacy appears a relatively widespread, if mostly temporary phenomenon, on the eve of the industrial revolution. Flandrin's study (1979: p. 184) of French family and kinship patterns suggests similar trends: 'often the seduced girl was driven away as soon as the pregnancy became evident, and it was in isolation, in the country or in a big town, that she gave birth to and then abandoned her child.'

Foundling Hospitals were set up to look after babies and children who might otherwise be killed or abandoned in the fields or streets. Many of the mothers were single women but not all – child-bearing was an expensive business and many married couples could not afford an extra mouth to feed. One of the first Foundling Hospitals was set up in 1741 in London by Thomas Coram (see Hibbert 1987). In 1756, the hospital was opened to children all over the country and this led to a deluge of babies and children being left on its doorstep. About 10,000 children died in the hospital between 1756 to 1800 owing to the excessive numbers and poor condition of the children it was being asked to deal with. Restrictions were then made to the types of children that might be admitted. Only the first children of unmarried mothers would be accepted; the fathers must have deserted the mother and child; and the mother must have been of good repute before her 'fall'.

A particular difficulty with historical data on the family is that most data pertain to the upper and middle classes. And it is among these classes that marriage and legitimacy were most important (owing to the need to secure the correct inheritance of property rights). Evidence suggests that informal unions and illegitimacy were much more acceptable and widespread among the poor and the working class. The link between illegitimacy and poverty is suggested by Houlbrooke (1984) who quotes that a third of all illegitimate births in the village of Terling between 1570 and 1699 occurred in just one decade – 1597–1607. His explanation for this is that many people postponed wedding plans due to a run of bad harvests during that decade.

Industrialisation, Victorian values and the 'era of mandatory marriage'

The diversity in family patterns which existed particularly among the working classes began to die away from the mid-eighteenth century onwards. By the mid-nineteenth century, informal marriage customs were rare and illegitimacy more widely stigmatised. Gillis labels the period from 1850 to 1960 'the era of mandatory marriage'. Traditional practices which allowed a degree of sexual nonconformity were becoming increasingly rare as Victorian respectability placed a stranglehold on personal sexual liberty.

Cohabitation and illegitimacy declined. But they were not wiped out completely and women often suffered as a consequence. The 1834 Poor Law reforms defined women's rights to welfare according to strict patriarchal principles. Gillis states (1985: p. 239) that: 'The clauses with respect to bastardy were among the harshest of the entire 1834 code. Unwed mothers were stripped of their right to outdoor relief.' Lone mothers were struggling to manage and the number of children abandoned to Foundling Hospitals and orphanages increased.

Why did people in the early nineteenth century begin to conform to laws they had ignored or resisted for decades? Gillis (1985: p. 241/2) points to two explanations. First: 'a century of moral vigilance campaigns' which were run by the propertied classes to impose their values on the rest of society. Second, and more importantly, the 'evolution of industrial capitalism which . . . consigned to men the role of principal breadwinner and to women the destiny of dependent wife and mother'. Women's share of paid work declined during the nineteenth century, giving them less economic freedom and forcing them into greater dependence on men. Another consequence of industrialisation and urbanisation was that when a single woman became pregnant it was more difficult for her to prove who the father was because of the greater anonymity of the city compared with the village or small town. But while cohabitation and illegitimacy declined, the ideal of conjugal love and 'happy ever after' failed to become a lived reality for the majority.

Victorian culture combined with (or was perhaps produced by) the imperatives of industrialisation to introduce new conventions in family life. A strict moral code was established that people were expected to adhere to. Husband and wife were seen as one, or rather the wife was subsumed within the husband. The husband was quite clearly the head of the household. For example, the wife had no right to her own property until the Acts of the 1870s and 1880s. Duty rather than love or personal satisfaction was seen as the basis of marriage at that time. However, divorce was made slightly more possible by an Act in 1857 and between 1859 and 1909, there were 17,952 divorces – about 350 a year (Kiernan et al. 1998). Divorce was still heavily stigmatised, however, and only an option for the richest. Separation – both informal and legalised after the 1878 Matrimonial Causes Act – was more common with 6,559 legal separations occurring in 1907 alone (Kiernan et al. 1998).

The Victorian era saw the ascendancy of the married nuclear family but there were some trends to the contrary. For example, the anonymity found in the new towns and cities allowed some people to act in a way that would have attracted stigma and disgrace in a small rural community.

Men, in particular, could abandon wives in large towns and cities (or perhaps abandon them in the country and then go to the new urban areas) and could escape the censure of the people around them. And death rates among the poor were high. Rowntree's study of poverty in York at the turn of the twentieth century estimated that 16 per cent of all poor people were widows (Rowntree 1901). But divorce and illegitimacy became more heavily frowned on and the early twentieth century saw a growing emphasis on the importance of the nuclear family.

The first half of the twentieth century to some extent saw a continuation of Victorian values and practices but there were also some signs of a challenge to this way of life. Pedersen (1993: p. 132) has investigated this period from the point of view of family policy and found that 'in Britain . . . the [First World] war strengthened a particular conception of the family and gave rise to new campaigns determined to incorporate that vision into state policy itself.' In Britain, however, the war left some women with the right to vote and 'first wave' feminists such as Eleanor Rathbone were determined to fight for the rights of women (as housewives) to a secure and independent income. In 1918, the National Council for the Unmarried Mother and her Child was established to campaign on behalf of this group (it subsequently became the National Council for One Parent Families and still campaigns today). The 1920s saw the promotion of ideas of 'free love' by Bertrand Russell and others. Birth control was also being hailed as a means of separating sex from marriage and child-bearing.

The dominance of Victorian values in the early part of the twentieth century was therefore great but such values were beginning to be challenged. The depression of the 1930s, however, saw the decline of radical ideas and the focus of the British government was on the (male) unemployed rather than the housewife. Policy was based once again around the patriarchal nuclear family.

The heyday of Victorian values actually occurred about half a century after Victoria died. During the 1950s there were very low rates of illegitimacy and separation/divorce. The middle class nuclear family became the established norm from which few deviated. But the triumph of this particular family form was to be relatively short-lived.

The second half of the twentieth century: a return to informality and diversity?

The Second World War saw women moving into the factories and the farms as workers. The divorce and illegitimacy rates rose. But the end of the war saw the promotion once again of the nuclear family, motherhood and child-bearing. Evidence suggests that most men and women were happy to return to their gendered roles after the chaos of war. Kiernan *et al.* (1998) suggest that cohabitation was probably rarer in the 1950s and 1960s than it was at the turn of the twentieth century. The divorce rate was also low. Studies at the time showed that the majority of women were virgins when they married and bridal virginity was seen as heavily prized by men (Roberts 1995). Children lived with their parents until they married and so had little opportunity for sexual activity with boyfriends or girl-friends. Those that did have sex and got pregnant faced shame and stigma and were often forced into 'shotgun weddings'.

The 1960s is sometimes referred to as the permissive era or the 'swinging sixties' but such permissiveness was probably experienced only by a very few. Birth control was slowly becoming more easily available – both in the form of condoms and the contraceptive pill – owing to the 1967 Family Planning Act. The 1967 Abortion Act made certain forms of abortion legal and the 1969 legislation on divorce made divorce much easier for people from all walks of life. A self-help group for lone parents, Gingerbread, was launched in 1970 and grew from strength to strength. The patriarchal model of marriage and the family was beginning to be questioned. In relation to women, Gummer (1971: p. 24) lamented that 'the whole concept of courtship and capture has been broken down.' Personal satisfaction and partnership rather than romance and duty came to be seen as the basis for a new model of married life (see below). The explanation for these changes is often discussed in terms of the emerging economic, political, social and cultural power of 'youth' (Evans 1993). Whatever the causes and extent of 'permissiveness' the 1960s sowed the seeds of changing attitudes and behaviour but the fruit of these changes was yet to emerge fully.

Changes in family life are closely linked to structural economic change and the 1970s saw the emergence of what has been termed 'post-industrialisation'. The recession of the late 1970s brought mass unemploy-ment to the UK for the first time since the 1930s and the economy was never the same again, with a terminal decline in basic industries such as coal, steel and ship-building as well as more general manufacturing. Service and financial industries emerged and new forms of employment, particularly part-time work, became more widespread. The decline of 'mandatory marriage' might be seen as accompanying the decline of industrialisation. Divorce increased dramatically, as did the number of lone parent families created through this route.

The 1980s appeared to usher in a new tide of individualism and self-interest both in economic and family life. After the recession of the early 1980s, the boom of the late 1980s saw an increase in conspicuous consumption and hedonism as individuals chased the high life. Inequality grew so that, while some enjoyed increases in incomes, others struggled more and more to make ends meet (Hills 1995). From the mid-1980s onwards, the 'permissive society' appeared to be in retreat with increasing concern about the spread of HIV. The introduction of Section 28 of the Local Government Act 1988 also had an impact as it forbade local authorities to 'promote' homosexuality. And there was also the Gillick case in 1986 that sought to challenge the right of children under 16 to get confidential contraceptive advice from their doctors. This decade saw the continued growth in the number of separated and divorced lone parents but a relatively new phenomenon also emerged – the growth of single, never-married lone mothers.

As we shall see in the next section of this chapter, the late twentieth century witnessed major change in family structures and demographic forms. Lone parenthood should therefore be seen in the context of more general demographic change. People are cohabiting rather than, or in advance of, getting married. They are getting married and having children at later ages than in the 1950s and 1960s. They are having fewer children and more are not having any children at all. They are also more likely to get divorced and re-marry, leading to a rise in the number of step-families. People are also more likely than before to live on their own, particularly if they are older people, owing to the lengthening of life-spans, but there has also been a rise in the number of younger people who are single and living alone. The changes here are seen as so fundamental that some demographers refer to them as the 'second demographic transition' (Coleman and Chandola 1999).

Changes in family structures, accompanied by social and economic change, have also led to changes in relationships *within* the family – between women and men, between parents and children, and between adults and their parents. The 'breadwinner/housewife' model which reached its peak in the 1950s is far less common today. This is due partly to the rise of lone parenthood but, even among couples with children, the woman is quite likely to be in employment, at least part-time. The increase in numbers of absent fathers and step-families has changed the relationships between parents and children such that biological ties have been loosened from social ties, even if organisations such as the Child Support Agency are trying to enforce obligations based on past biological associations rather than current personal and/or socio-economic associations. The growth of lone parenthood has, in some cases, encouraged closer ties between adults and their parents (particularly between women and their mothers). Ties between adults and their parents have also been changing due to the age-ing of the population. People in middle age are increasingly confronting decisions about the care of their parents.

In this section we have seen that if we take a broad historical per-spective, the rise in cohabitation and lone parenthood appears more like a return to old traditions of self-marriage and self-divorce rather than a totally new form of family life. Similarly, growth in illegitimacy and lone parenthood does not appear to signify 'the death of the family'. It may signify the death of the nuclear family (though the word death is over-stating it). Another way of describing the changes is as a return to more diverse family patterns which were not uncommon before industrialisation.

2.2 The recent growth of lone parenthood

As discussed above, there has been a rapid increase in the number of lone parent families since 1970 (starting from a very low base in the 1950s and 1960s) (Haskey 1994). In 1971 there were 570,000 lone parents. Ten years later, this number had grown steadily to about 900,000. The rate of growth then slowed slightly over the next few years only to cross the one million mark by 1986. The rate of growth then picked up again to reach 1.4 million by 1992, and around 1.6 million by the late 1990s (Haskey 1998).

Official statistics also show that lone parenthood grew faster than the overall growth in the number of households or of the number of fam-ilies with children. For example, in 1971, only 3 per cent of *all households* were lone parent households, according to the General Household Survey. By 1994, this figure had risen to 7 per cent and was 9 per cent in 1997/98. Among *families* with dependent children, lone parents accounted for 8 per cent in 1971. This figure almost tripled by 1994 so that almost a quarter (23 per cent) of all families with children in 1994 were headed by a lone parent. In 1972, 6 per cent of children lived in a lone parent family. By 1994/95, this had increased to 20 per cent (Central Statistical Office 1996).

Throughout the 1970s, 1980s and 1990s, about nine lone parents in ten were women. Lone fatherhood is not a very widespread phenom-enon and has become a smaller component of lone parenthood in the last 20 years. In 1971, there were 70,000 lone fathers – 13 per cent of all lone parents (Haskey 1994). By 1991, there were 100,000 – 9 per cent of all lone parents. Some forms of child-sharing arrangements may, how-ever, become increasingly important for fathers if their relationships break down.

The majority of lone mothers in the 1970s, 1980s and 1990s had separated or divorced from their spouse. A smaller, though increasing group, were single, never-married women with children. It is important to note, however (as discussed in Chapter 1), that most official statistics rely heavily on legal marital status to define lone mothers and this means that women who have had children with a cohabiting partner and then separate from him are classified as single, never-married lone mothers, along with single women who have never cohabited but have a baby. The growth of cohabitation in the last 20 or so years therefore exaggerates the growth in the number of single women who have babies outside a steady partnership.

In the 1970s, the proportion of lone parents who had separated or divorced from their spouses rose faster than other groups. In the early 1980s, separated/divorced women continued to be an increasingly important component of lone parenthood but in the late 1980s and early 1990s, the proportion of separated lone parents tailed off slightly, giving way to a rapid growth in the proportion of lone parents who were single, never-married mothers.

The number of widowed lone parents has declined since the 1970s. In 1971, there were 120,000 widowed lone parents (Haskey 1994). By 1976, this number had fallen slightly to 115,000 and by 1986, this number had fallen more substantially to about 70,000, where it has remained, more or less, ever since (Haskey 1994). Widowed lone parents tend to be older and have older children than other lone parents. In Britain, widows have generally received more favourable treatment in social security policy compared with other lone parents. They are also firmly on the side of the line marked 'deserving' as they cannot (usually) be held 'responsible' for having become a lone parent. Widowed lone parents are therefore more likely to receive sympathy than blame or stigma.

2.3 Explaining the recent growth of lone parenthood

The recent growth of lone parenthood has been rather rapid and has caused concern among some politicians, policy-makers and members of the public. So why did it happen? There is no uncontested theory to explain the recent rise in lone parenthood but a number of factors are put forward as possible contributory causes including:

● Changes in the overall and relative employment prospects of men and women.

- Changes in the availability of social security and housing.

- Changes in divorce legislation and attitudes to divorce.

- Changes in sexual attitudes and behaviour, including changes in availability of contraception and abortion.

- Changes in attitudes to 'the family'and the individual.

- The rise of feminist ideas and increasing intolerance of male domination and violence.

Each of these factors could have an effect on:

- The number of single women who have children.

- The number of women with children who separate from partners.

- The length of time women remain as lone parents.

We briefly review some of the current evidence for these explanations.

Employment prospects of men and women

Since the 1960s, there has been a rise in the proportion of women who are in paid employment, particularly those in the middle of their working lives. Over a similar period, there has been a dramatic decline in male employment, particularly among men at both ends of the age distribution. According to the Labour Force Survey, the employment rate for men of working age was 94 per cent in 1959 compared with 79 per cent in 1999 and the decline was much more significant for men in their teenage years and early 20s. Among women, the figures are 47 per cent employment rate in 1959 and 69 per cent in 1999 (Office of National Statistics 2001). If we focus on women in particular age groups – in this case their late 20s and early 30s, the changes are much more pronounced. And the main changes for women have occurred among those who are married and, even more so, those who are married and have young children. In 1977–79, only about a quarter (27 per cent) of married women with children under 5 were in paid work. By 1992–94, the proportion had risen to a half (51 per cent) (Central Statistical Office 1996). Most of these women are working part-time but about a third of them are working full-time. So there have been considerable changes in the relative labour market experiences of men and women, especially in relation to family formation issues.

American researchers have argued that the major factor underlying the growth of lone parenthood is the shift in the relative earnings opportunities of men and women. They argue that this affects poor people (mostly black people) in differently from better-off people (mostly whites). For poorer groups/black people, male unemployment not only reduces the economic incentive for women to marry but it also undermines the role of the husband as breadwinner. Hence it causes marital breakdown and reduces the likelihood that lone parents (or unmarried pregnant teenagers) will marry. For better-off groups/white people, the growth of lone parenthood is explained by the dramatic increase in labour force participation of women, which accelerated after the Second World War and has continued ever since. By working and earning more, women have achieved greater economic independence, which has reduced the costs of being single and increased the likelihood of experiencing marital breakdown (Garfinkel and McLanahan 1986: p. 167).

In the USA, lone parents are much more likely to be ethnic minorities than in Britain. We would argue that there are similar underlying causes of lone parenthood in Britain (lack of 'marriageable men' and so on) but that the issue of class is the more pertinent issue here rather than ethnicity.

Changes in the labour market and in the relative economic prospects of young men and women could have various effects on the growth of lone parenthood. For example, they could:

● increase conflict within marriage as traditional gender roles break down (e.g. because women are less keen to do (all the) unpaid work in the home after a day in their paid job);

● enable women in unhappy relationships to feel they have enough economic independence to leave their partners;

● increase the opportunities for both men and women to find other partners (at work) or to have extra-marital affairs which could lead to relationship breakdown;

● enable women in well-paid jobs to afford to have a baby without a partner;

● reduce the attraction of young single men as potential breadwinners and therefore encourage young single women to have children without cohabiting with the fathers;

● enable lone parents to support their families though employment thus reducing the need to find a partner who is a breadwinner.

While some women have benefited from their increasing employment opportunities, those with low educational achievement are likely to be facing the prospect of a life in a low-paid service sector job. Compared with such a future, the prospect of becoming a mother and looking after a child might seem appealing. It is therefore important that we do not simply take a gendered perspective on changing employment opportunities. Some women are benefiting from these changes but others may not be, likewise men. The effects of changing employment opportunities are therefore complex and vary depending on gender and social class but they are probably key factors in explaining the growth of lone parenthood.

The availability of social security and housing

As argued in Chapter 1, it has become widely believed, even among lone parents themselves, that some women become lone mothers because they know that they will receive social security benefits and a home from the state for simply being a lone parent (see Chapters 5 and 9 for further discussion of these issues).

But there have been social security benefits for lone parents ever since the Second World War and so the existence of social security and social housing, in themselves, have not led to the growth of lone parenthood. Marsden (1969), however, argued that although social security benefits were available to lone parents in the 1960s, there was a conspiracy of silence surrounding information about their availability. There is certainly no such conspiracy today. But, regardless of levels of knowledge, what may have changed is the acceptability of claiming benefit as a lone parent and the increasing scarcity of subsidised accommodation.

Although lone parents have been able to claim benefits for many years, there have been some changes in recent years which may have made a difference. For example, the 1988 Fowler reforms generally targeted benefits towards families with children and so could be seen as encouraging (lone) parenthood. Also, 16–17-year-olds are entitled to benefits only in certain circumstances, one of which is being a lone parent. So lone parenthood may be one of the few options for young women to set up a home independently from their parents and/or any partner.

There is also some concern in government that social security benefits for lone parents are more generous than those for couples. This apparent incentive to be a lone parent was addressed in 1997 by abolishing One Parent Benefit and the lone parent premium in means-tested benefits. Research, however, suggests that the benefit system is not generous to lone parents as it finds that couples can live as cheaply as (if not more cheaply than) single people (Berthoud and Ford 1996).

As mentioned above, social housing is becoming increasingly scarce and one way of being a priority on a housing list is to have children – whether with a partner or not (although there have been some moves to change this). If we put all these changes together then lone parenthood may be a relatively attractive option for young women from poor backgrounds.

As discussed in Chapter 1, however, comparative research (Whiteford and Bradshaw, 1994) suggests that social security systems, while treating lone parents in different ways, do not appear to affect behaviour towards becoming a lone parent.

Hoynes (1996) reviews a number of studies in the USA and comes to a similar conclusion that: 'the evidence suggests that family structure decisions are not sensitive to financial incentives'. She makes the important point that there has been a dramatic decline in the value of social assistance benefits in the USA since the 1960s – the very period during which the number of lone parent families increased and the number of births to single women increased.

Divorce law

There is a strong popular view that liberal divorce laws do not just facilitate divorce, they encourage people to divorce who would not otherwise do so. The evidence shows that there was an increase in divorces in the 1970s soon after the 1969 Divorce Act came into effect in 1971. However, there had also been some increase in divorce in the late 1960s. So an increase in the number of divorces probably led to the Act rather than vice versa. It is probably true that the Act made it easier for people who wanted to divorce to do so and as a result the number of divorces probably did also increase as a result of the law. But it is more difficult to argue that the Act would have encouraged people to separate.

In the USA, more than half of all the states had enacted some form of no-fault divorce legislation in the 1970s (beginning with California in 1970). Divorce statistics, however, show that the rates of divorce were no higher in these states than would be expected from the trend in states that had not reformed their laws (Wright and Stetson 1978). So the introduction of no-fault divorce should be seen as a reaction to changing attitudes and behaviour rather than a cause of such changes.

Sexual attitudes and behaviour

There have been significant changes in sexual attitudes and behaviour over the last 20 to 30 years that may have led to an increase in lone parenthood. For example, people are starting to have sexual intercourse at younger ages and this may increase the chances that a single woman will get pregnant (Wellings *et al.* 1994). However, the increasing availability of contraception in the form of the pill from the late 1960s onwards was supposed to free women from the fear of unwanted pregnancy, so the wider incidence of pre-marital sex, on its own, cannot account for the growth in single lone parenthood. The availability of contraceptive technology, however, is not sufficient on its own to guarantee its successful use. The Social Exclusion Unit's (1999) report on teenage pregnancy stresses the ignorance of many young people about contraception, sexually transmitted infections, pregnancy and so on. It is this ignorance that can explain some of the unplanned and unwanted pregnancies of single women.

Blake and Das Gupta (1975) have shown that economic conditions, social attitudes and motivations to either conceive or avoid conception, play an important role, and are perhaps more important than the availability of contraception.

Accidental pregnancies can, in theory, be terminated. Abortion became legal in Britain in 1968 and while the law does not allow abortion simply 'on demand' there is a great deal of discretion that doctors may apply. Rates of abortion are fairly high but availability is only the first step on the road to having an abortion – social attitudes will also play a major part, as will knowledge about abortion and access to services. About a third of all conceptions outside marriage ended in abortion in 1997 (Population Trends 1999).

Conceptions outside marriage do not necessarily lead to the creation of a lone parent family. As we have seen, some of these pregnancies are terminated. Others might lead to a birth within marriage if the parents marry each other. In the past, such 'shotgun weddings' may have been common, but in 1997 only 6 per cent of all conceptions outside marriage led to births within marriage. A total of six in ten conceptions outside marriage in 1997 led to births outside marriage. But many of these would have been to cohabiting couples. It is difficult to get accurate figures on this but we do know that only one in ten conceptions outside marriage was registered solely by the mother (Population Trends 1999). This does not necessarily mean that she was living alone but is an indicator of such.

An interesting and difficult question arises about how attitudinal change occurs. One way of answering this question is to take either an explicitly or implicitly structuralist approach and argue that attitudinal change is the result of changing economic and social structures, such as those in the labour market. This approach leaves very little room for individual agency: the ability of individuals to consciously reflect on their lives and make decisions to change their future. An alternative approach would be to see people as the conscious agents of change, not merely individuals who respond, in an apparently automatic fashion, to external forces. As we shall see, Giddens (1991, 1992) has been one of the main proponents of an agency approach, particularly in the field of personal relationships.

Attitudes to 'the family' and individual happiness

It has been argued that the growth of individualism can account for both the growth of the nuclear family in the 1950s and its decline in later parts of the twentieth century. It is argued that the nineteenth-century extended family was progressively destroyed by the growth of individualism which led, in the 1950s, to the promotion of a smaller family unit – the nuclear family. But the spread of the individualistic ethos did not stop there and has progressed to destroy the nuclear family, this time in favour of lone parent families and people living on their own. It is argued that individual happiness is now promoted rather than the good of the community, the extended family or the nuclear family.

Ingelhart (1977, 1990) has argued that there has been a shift from conservative values emphasising duty, responsibility and order to values emphasising self-realisation and autonomy. This shift from a value system emphasising obligations to others, religious duty and respect for traditional authority towards a value system promoting individualised rights and personal self-fulfilment has, it is argued, affected both women's and men's attitudes and feelings of obligations towards partners and children. Thus culture and identity are also likely to be important factors driving the growth of lone parenthood.

Giddens (1992) argues that people are now searching for a 'pure relationship' which is based on mutual, individual satisfaction and is the result of negotiation between two people. He also puts forward the idea that 'confluent love' has taken the place of romantic love in as much as people are interested in active, contingent love which does not necessarily last forever. Thus couples are more likely to split up if their partnership does not meet the ideal of a 'pure relationship' and relationships owe more to lifestyle choice than feelings of duty or obligation. Giddens, however, seems to be focusing mainly on people without children and says little about whether the presence of children affects feelings of duty or decisions to separate.

Beck and Beck-Gernsheim (1995) make the interesting (and seemingly contradictory) point that the growth of individualism in late modernity has resulted in people yearning for close relationships with others. They argue that this desperate need for love is now focusing more on children as love between adults has become so unreliable and contingent. This is evident in the number of single women who are willing to have children without a partner and the number of men who wish to retain relationships with their children even though their partnership with the mother has ended.

Attitudes to relationships, marriage and lone parenthood have certainly changed over the last 50 years. But, as mentioned above, it is difficult to know whether such attitudinal changes were the cause or effect of changes in behaviour. Studies have tended to show that attitudes to the family have followed rather than led to changes in behaviour (Cherlin 1992). For example, opinion poll data in the USA have shown that attitudes to divorce did not begin to change noticeably until about 1970 whereas the increase in divorce rates began in the mid to late 1960s. But although these changes in attitude were not the initial driving force for changes in behaviour they may have fed back into a second round, or second generation, of behavioural changes (Cherlin 1992), leading to a spiralling of changes.

Further evidence of the relationship between attitudes and behaviour comes from an American panel study which involved interviews with 900 young, white mothers. These women were interviewed between 1962 and 1977. Those who had originally agreed with the statement: 'when there are children in the family, parents should stay together even if they don't get along', were only slightly less likely to be separated or divorced by the end of the study period than those who had disagreed with it. So their attitudes to the family appear to have had little impact on their behaviour. However, their behaviour then had an impact on their attitudes – those who had separated or divorced by the end of the study period were much less likely to agree with the statement subsequently (Thornton 1985).

The rise of feminism and increasing intolerance of male domination and violence

The women's movement from the 1970s onwards has no doubt played a role in relation to the rise of lone parenthood. The women's movement has fought for a better deal for women in employment, social security, access to abortion and contraception. It has also played a part in arguing for more sexual freedom for women and autonomy from men in general. As argued in the next chapter, feminism has many strands and it is difficult to link the rise of the women's movement directly to the rise of lone parenthood: some aspects of the women's movement might be thought to lead to a reduction in lone parenthood (such as the fight for increased abortion and contraception rights); other aspects might be thought to lead to a rise in lone parenthood (such as the demand for greater autonomy from men). Whatever the precise nature of the relationship, feminist thought has played an important role at a time when numbers of lone parents have been on the increase. At the very least it has provided a source of support for lone mothers.

There is one area in particular in which feminist ideals seem to have played a key role. This is in relation to the issue of domestic violence. Before the rise of the women's movement in the 1970s, wives of violent men had little option but to stay put. The police were reluctant to get involved in 'private' matters between husband and wife and there was little material support (in terms of alternative accommodation) that a woman could draw on. Indeed, social services tried to encourage 'problem families' to stay together unless the children were being directly abused. In the 1970s, however, things began to change. The Women's Aid Federations began to set up refuges. These not only provided practical support for women to leave their abusive partners but also became symbolic beacons to tell society that domestic violence was unacceptable. In the 1980s, police procedures on domestic violence received widespread criticism. This led to Home Office circular 60/90 in 1990 which emphasised the need for dedicated units and specialist officers, clear strategies for dealing with domestic violence and the presumption of arrest where an offence had been committed. However, by the late 1990s not all police forces had implemented these recommendations (Plotnikoff and Woolfson 1998). And even if they had, Grace (1995) has argued that policy implementation does not guarantee good practice.

There is much less tolerance for domestic violence today than there was in the 1950s and 1960s, not least because of concern for children in violent homes. Research has found that domestic violence is correlated, to some extent, with child abuse. And even where children are not directly being abused, they suffer in a range of ways (physically, emotionally, educationally and so on) from being in a violent home (Morley and Mullender 1994).

More and more mothers appear to be leaving violent partners. Cockett and Tripp (1994) found that one in four separated women with children had separated from their partners due to domestic violence. Marsh *et al.* (2001) found that a third of all lone parents with former partners (excluding widows) said that during their last year together some of their arguments had led to physical violence.

We might think and hope that domestic violence, as a result of changing attitudes, is a thing of the past. Unfortunately it remains. According to Mirrlees-Black (1999) 23 per cent of women and 15 per cent of men aged 16–59 said that they had been physically assaulted by a partner at some point in the past. Female victims were more likely than male victims to experience more severe forms of violence. Female victims were more likely to be young women, not in paid work, on a low income and mothers (a profile not dissimilar to lone mothers). Of victims who had children, about a third said that the children had been aware of the last assault. The researchers estimated that in 1995 there had been 6.6 million incidents of domestic violence (including 2.9 million incidents of injury) and a further 7 million incidents of frightening threats.

2.4 Summary

During the first half of the twentieth century, lone parenthood was relatively rare and was confined mostly to widows. The last 30 years of the twentieth century saw a dramatic rise in the number of lone parents and this has concerned some commentators who bemoan the 'death of the family'. However, if we take a longer look in history we find that, prior to industrialisation, lone parenthood and cohabitation were much more common than in the middle of the twentieth century. It is probably the 1950s, and early 1960s, that stand out as unusual historically with stable families and secure male employment.

Until the middle of the eighteenth century, lone parenthood was relatively common. Widowhood was a common cause of lone parenthood, though the prospects of severe hardship led many women re-partner after a suitable period of mourning (usually about a year). Some lone parent families were formed at this time owing to women separating from their husbands.

While it is difficult to draw firm conclusions from relatively scant empirical evidence, it has been argued that formal marriage and the nuclear family should be seen as the experiment rather than the universal norm. Pre-industrial society certainly seems to be characterised by informal and shifting relationships rather than long-term, formal, stable nuclear family structures.

The advent of industrialisation, however, began to change this. Hardwicke's Marriage Act of 1753 formalised secular marriage alongside religious ceremonies. A century later, informal marriage customs were rare and illegitimacy more widely stigmatised. The 1834 Poor Laws included harsh clauses to punish single motherhood. The number of children abandoned to orphanages increased.

During the late twentieth century family life became more diverse. Cohabitation, illegitimacy and divorce increased. Increasing numbers of women chose not to have children. More and more women, particularly mothers, joined (or re-joined) the labour market. There has been an increase in dual earner couples as well as no-earner couples. The bread-winner/housewife nuclear family model is no longer universal.

The 1970s and early 1980s saw an increase in the numbers of lone parent families and most of these were created when women separated and divorced from their husbands. In the late 1980s and 1990s, the increase in lone parenthood continued, this time fuelled most by women separating from cohabiting partners and by women having babies without partners at all. We have already seen that these patterns of family life are not new but why did they emerge in the last few decades of the twentieth century? A number of possible explanations emerge, including the following:

- Changing economic and employment patterns for both men and women.
- The availability of social security benefits and social housing for lone parents.
- Changing attitudes to sex, marriage and illegitimacy.
- Changing attitudes to the family and individual happiness.
- The rise of feminism and increasing intolerance of male domination and violence.

The rise of lone parenthood is a phenomenon that has occurred in most advanced industrial countries (though to varying extents). This suggests, along with historical evidence, that it is related to changes in the basic structure of social and economic life, and to changes in the way that people, women in particular, choose to live their lives. We are moving from an industrial world to a post-industrial world and the growth of lone parenthood is one part of this transition.

chapter 3

Thinking about lone parenthood

In Chapter 1 we analysed the situation of lone parent families today and in Chapter 2 we took a broader historical approach to lone parenthood. In this chapter we take a step back from the facts and figures on lone parenthood to consider different ways of conceptualising lone parenthood. But whereas there is a wealth of sociological theory surrounding *the family* in general, there is little relating specifically to lone parenthood. Such theoretical approaches might help us to understand different aspects of lone parenthood such as its growth in recent years, its place in contemporary society, the experiences of lone parents and so on. This chapter applies four general sociological theories to lone parenthood. These are functionalism, Marxism, feminism and post-modernism. It then focuses on class and gender to see how these concepts can aid our understanding of lone parenthood. Ideologies around parenthood and childhood are also pertinent to this book's theme and they are outlined in the following section. The chapter ends by discussing in detail the issues surrounding how we define lone parenthood.

3.1 Sociological approaches to the family

There are four main sociological approaches that can be usefully applied to an understanding of the family and lone parenthood. The first of these, *functionalism*, views society as a system of inter-related and inter-dependent parts (Parsons 1951). This general theoretical perspective therefore emphasises stability and coherence. Each part of society is seen as providing some necessary social function (or need) and thus contributing to the maintenance and integration of the society as a whole. One consequence of this inter-connectedness is that change in any one part of society will affect other parts, but generally through a slow process of evolution rather than through any sudden or violent revolution. The family, which in functionalist terms is usually defined as the nuclear family, is therefore considered in terms of the functions it performs and the relationships it has with other social institutions. Broadly speaking, the nuclear family is seen as fulfilling the basic social need for the regulation of sexual behaviour and for the conception, care and socialisation of children. Functionalists tend to see the family as maintaining the overall stability and harmony of society.

Functionalism became popularised in the 1950s through the work of the American sociologist, Talcott Parsons. It was based on a particular picture of society at that time, in which mothers stayed at home to look after children while their breadwinning husbands went out to work. Such a system of 'teamwork' was considered by functionalists to be highly important in maintaining social stability and integration (Parsons and Bales 1956). A functionalist approach to lone parenthood would be critical of the institution, seeing it as dysfunctional in some ways. The ability of lone parents to socialise their children adequately would be questioned. Functionalists might also have concerns about the stability of a society with substantial numbers of lone parents. Those who argued that the twentieth century was in danger of witnessing the 'death of the family' were usually arguing from a functionalist perspective.

Marxism is the second general sociological theory that can be usefully applied to the family. Marxist theory shares some similarities with functionalism but is, in many ways, radically different. Rather than seeing society as a series of inter-related parts, Karl Marx effectively saw society as divided between an economic 'base' (the mode of production and the relations of production) and a 'superstructure' (including political and legal institutions). The economic base was considered to be the engine of social change, while the superstructure evolved as a consequence of initial changes in the base. Thus changes in the family (which form part of the superstructure) would be the consequence of changes in the economic base. Marx also saw society in terms of conflict, with capitalist society characterised by class conflict between workers and owners of the means of production. Thus change would not come about through peaceful, evolutionary means but through violent, sudden revolution (Marx and Engels [1849] 1934). Karl Marx himself paid little attention to the family as he saw it as largely a peripheral issue. Engels, however, developed his own ideas on the subject. He explored the role of the monogamous nuclear family as a means of transmitting property from one generation to another (Engels 1972). Lone parent families might, therefore, be seen as a challenge to patriarchal forms of capitalism. As we shall see, Marxist feminists have applied a Marxist perspective to gender relations and family life.

While functionalism and Marxism tend to take a male-centred approach to social questions, *feminist theorists* have put women back into the picture. Feminist theorists have traditionally been classified as liberal, Marxist or radical/separatist but this classification has itself been criticised for over-simplifying the diversity of feminist thought. It also misses out some key strands of thought such as psychoanalytical feminism and newer forms of feminism drawing on post-modernist approaches (Stacey 1993). Having said all this, it is worth broadly reviewing Marxist feminism and radical feminism as they have distinct approaches to gender inequality and the family.

In broad terms, Marxist feminists argue that women's subordinate position in capitalist society is due to their relationship to the world of paid employment. Women have been side-lined from the world of paid employment so that they can reproduce the labour force through the care and socialisation of children. They can also be considered a reserve army of labour (Barrett 1980). Some Marxist feminists consider the working class family as providing a source of support and solidarity in a conflictual world. Radical feminists argue that women's subordinate position is due to the patriarchal power that men exercise over women in most societies, regardless of the nature of the economy or employment (Firestone 1971, Millett 1971). While Marxist feminists consider both class and gender as important aspects of socio-economic division, radical feminists consider gender to be of primary, if not sole, importance. Radical feminists see the nuclear family as an institution that serves to oppress women through securing unpaid personal and domestic services as well as socialising girls and boys into their gender-designated roles. These theorists might therefore consider lone parents as pioneers in the struggle against the patriarchal institution of the nuclear family. Some feminists view lone parenthood as a challenge to private patriarchy (the domination of women by men in the home). But the dependence of lone parents on the state might be seen as a form of public patriarchy.

Post-modernist theorists challenge all grand narratives including those relating to capitalism and patriarchy (Lyotard 1984). They stress the diversity of social experience and criticise the notion of collectivities such as class and gender. Their analysis of class and gender is purely in terms of deconstructing these linguistic categories rather than analysing inequality or oppression. The key post-modern and post-structuralist theorists such as Foucault and Lyotard have paid little attention to gender and their ideas challenge the basic Marxist and feminist ideas that place class and gender as sites of oppression. Nevertheless many feminists have embraced the new approach to social issues (Barrett and Phillips 1992). This is partly because post-modernism takes a critical stance towards 'objectivity' in a similar way as feminist researchers have done. And the new way of seeing the complexity of power relations allows more sophisticated analysis of the experiences of different women. Some women are more powerful than others (and more powerful than some men). Women are different from each other in many ways and the recognition of this can be seen as an advance over the simplistic feminist view that all power rests with men, leaving women as mere passive victims rather than active agents. But while post-modernism and post-structuralism provide some positive avenues for feminist analysis, there is a danger of over-stressing difference and losing any notion of the importance of gender and class structures.

Duncan and Edwards (1999) have drawn on a post-modernist approach to apply a discourse analysis to lone motherhood. They identify four overlapping discourses around lone motherhood, as shown in Box 3.1. The 'social threat' and 'social problem' discourses are similar in that they both see lone motherhood as problematic but one takes a harsh view of the women themselves and the other takes a more sympathetic view. The 'lifestyle change' discourse is rather neutral about whether lone parenthood is a good thing or not. It argues that this is the way things are going and is the result of people making (rational) choices about how to live their lives. This is similar to the view mentioned above that lone parenthood is related to the growth of individualism and individual choice over lifestyle. The 'escaping patriarchy' discourse is the kind that radical feminists might follow. It takes a positive view of lone parenthood.

There are a number of issues relating to this (and any other) discourse analysis. It refuses to make any judgement about the relative validity of different discourses, merely seeking to describe them. However, the discourses outlined above contain some statements about lone parents that are empirically testable. It is therefore possible, to some extent, to see which discourse is most valid.

Bradley (1996: p. 3) argues that post-modernist approaches 'sit uneasily with study of material factors such as inequality and deprivation'. But she argues that this need not necessarily be the case. She calls for links to be made between 'materiality and meaning' as people with command of material resources generally have greatest power to define meaning and to shape the dominant discourse. Applying this to Duncan and Edwards' (1999)

Box 3.1 Four discourses on lone motherhood according to Duncan and Edwards (1999)

Lone parents as a **social threat**

Lone parents:

- are caused by welfare and feminism;
- choose to have children to get benefits and housing;
- don't want to work;
- are promiscuous;
- produce delinquent boys and promiscuous girls owing to lack of a father;
- wreck society.

Lone parents as a **social problem**

Lone parents:

- are victims needing help;
- are economically and socially disadvantaged;
- want to work but can't owing to poverty trap and childcare costs;
- produce delinquent boys and promiscuous girls owing to lack of a father.

Lone parents as **escaping patriarchy**

Lone mothers:

- don't want to be controlled by men;
- find it difficult to find 'new men';
- enjoy financial and emotional advantages over other women.

Lone parents as a reflection of **lifestyle change**

Lone mothers:

- make a choice out of many family forms;
- are a sign of future trends;
- are caused by a lack of breadwinning men;
- have a right to work and to divorce.

list of discourses, certain discourses will be more dominant than others because it is in the interests of the powerful to promote them. In recent years, the social threat discourse has been heavily promoted by politicians and the media.

The growth of individualism (as noted in Chapter 2) is sometimes seen as part of the move to a post-modern society (Ingelhart 1977). Old values, rules and ideas of morality are breaking down such that people can pick and choose their own lifestyles and living arrangements. It is within this context that Giddens (1992) and Beck and Beck-Gernsheim (1995) have written their influential books (see Chapter 2 for further discussion of their work). Giddens hardly uses the term 'family' but refers instead to how individuals feel and behave in relation to others. This signals the difficulties in defining 'the family' at a time when people live their lives in such diverse ways. It also signals the decreasing significance of 'the nuclear family' as an institution. Thus, in Giddens' framework, lone parenthood might be seen as an equally valid lifestyle choice as any other. The work of Giddens and Beck and Beck-Gernsheim has influenced recent research into, and thinking about, family life (Silva and Smart 1999, Smart and Neale 1999).

3.2 Gender and class perspectives on lone parenthood

Following on from feminist perspectives, the gender dimension of lone parenthood is the one most commonly applied:

> Single motherhood is a gendered position, shaped by notions of appropriate relationships between men and women and the roles of mothers and fathers.   (Duncan and Edwards 1997: p. 1)

And this perspective is most often applied in relation to lone parent poverty:

> It is precisely because lone mothers are women that they have a very high risk of poverty.   (Millar 1992: p. 149)

Millar (1992: p. 149) argues that the economic position of lone mothers must be analysed in the context of the economic position of women in general and this is the *only* way to understand the causes of their poverty. This is because the main source of economic power is via the labour market and women in general suffer from disproportionate access to the labour market. Millar and Glendinning (1992) argue that women are defined as 'secondary workers' in three ways. First, the paid work they do is considered to be secondary to their roles as domestic workers. They are therefore expected to give up paid work when it conflicts with their domestic responsibilities (and this unpaid work in the home is also valued very little). Second, women's work is considered secondary to men's. Third, even when they participate in the labour market they are often confined to the 'secondary' or 'peripheral' labour market, where the worst jobs are in terms of pay and conditions.

Women are also disadvantaged in relation to the social security system. Social security systems were generally established with the male

worker in mind. National Insurance benefits were designed to compens-
ate for periods out of the labour market due to sickness, unemployment
and retirement. Women often fail to accrue sufficient credits to take
advantage of these benefits. And in any case, their absence from the labour
market is more likely to be due to pregnancy and caring rather than
sickness and unemployment. Yet these contingencies are inadequately
covered by social security systems, particularly in the UK. Levels of means-
tested benefits are low in the UK and it is women who have the main
responsibility to make ends meet on them (see Chapter 5 for further
discussion).

It is clear that a gender approach to poverty is important in appreci-
ating how poverty affects women in general, and lone parents in particular.
Lone parents are disadvantaged because, as women, they are expected to
be the ones who look after their children in the home. Their access to the
labour market is restricted to secondary jobs and so many of them live on
inadequate levels of social security benefits.

But while the gender perspective is clearly central to an understanding
of lone parenthood it is not, we would argue, the 'only' way to understand lone parenthood. Other factors, such as ethnicity, disability, age and
so on are also important. This book emphasises the issue of social class.
The class dimension has received much less attention than gender for a
number of reasons:

- Feminist researchers are primarily interested in gender and it is
  these researchers who have paid attention to lone parenthood.

- Marxist researchers are primarily interested in class but they have
  not been particularly interested in either the family in general or
  lone parenthood in particular to date.

- The role of social class became much more complex in the second
  half of the twentieth century owing to changes in employment
  patterns. Increasing interest in post-modernist approaches has also
  sidelined 'essentialist' and structuralist concepts such as class and
  gender.

- Most classifications of social class use the occupation of the chief
  wage earner to categorise families. Most lone parents are not in
  paid work and so have no occupational status to use as a clear
  basis for class categorisation.

The class dimension has therefore been ignored partly due to lack
of interest and partly due to the difficulties in applying a class perspective. Nevertheless, a class dimension is illuminative and has indirectly

informed the debate around lone parenthood. Similarly, the rise of lone parenthood has affected the nature of social class in Britain. The 'traditional' class structure of the 1950s was the basis for the nuclear family that flourished at the same time. Changes in that class structure (in terms of the decline in male breadwinning jobs and the increase in female employment) have contributed to the rise of lone parenthood. Lone parents, particularly single lone mothers, are mostly women from poor working class backgrounds (see Chapter 1). Poverty and lack of opportunity are part of the reason why some single women become lone parents. The poor labour market status of potential husbands is also part of the picture. Equally poverty and unemployment can put strains on couples and cause some to split up. So while it is true that lone parenthood causes poverty, it is also the case that poverty causes lone parenthood. Lack of opportunities within the labour market is not just an issue of gender. During the 1980s and 1990s, young men and older men from working class backgrounds progressively dropped out of the labour market while middle class women formed an increasing part of the primary labour force.

Thus we could paraphrase the quote from Millar (1992) highlighted above. It is not simply the case that lone mothers are poor because they are women. It is also the case that poor women become lone mothers and remain poor or become even poorer. Of course some relatively wealthy women become lone mothers (Diana, Princess of Wales is a rather extreme example perhaps, but the example does show that lone parenthood is not simply confined to young women in inner city estates!). Middle class women who experience lone parenthood are likely to see their living standards reduced greatly – perhaps in some cases to a state of poverty. But the experiences of 'middle class' lone mothers are likely to be quite different from 'working class' lone mothers in terms of the resources they may be able to draw upon (for example in relation to housing, savings, maintenance, financial support from the extended family, labour market experience and so on). The lives of 'middle class' lone parents may be similar in some respects to those of 'working class' lone parents but they are also likely to be very different. We are therefore arguing that gender is an important factor in understanding lone parenthood but that other factors, class in particular, need similar attention.

People's lives are complex and it is almost impossible to analyse the relative importance of class, gender and other factors in explaining people's experiences. Nevertheless, it is important to be open to the range of factors that might be important rather than claiming that only one factor is at work.

3.3 Ideologies of parenthood and childhood

As well as looking at theories and conceptualisation in relation to the family, it is important to look at how ideologies of parenthood have been changing dramatically in recent decades. During the first half of the twentieth century, motherhood was considered to be an essential part of being a woman (Lewis 1980, Phoenix *et al.* 1991, Silva 1996). It was also considered to be inseparable from marriage. Women who could not have children were pitied and it was seldom considered possible that a woman might voluntarily choose not to have children. Once a woman had a child it was considered to be inevitable that she would devote her energies to caring for the child rather than doing a paid job. Today, motherhood is still generally considered central to a woman's life. But more women are choosing not to have children and so the apparently inseparable link between motherhood and womanhood is being challenged. It has been estimated that almost a quarter (23 per cent) of women born in 1974 will be childless when they reach 45 (in 2019) (Office of National Statistics 2001). Women without children might now be called 'child-free' as much as 'child-less' and this indicates a more positive view of life without children. Marriage is not now considered essential for motherhood (though it is still generally considered to be desirable). When women do have children they are less likely to give up work completely than they would have done in the past. Many might take on part-time work first (especially once the child goes to school) but it is increasingly rare for women to spend the whole of their lives as mothers outside the labour market.

There are numerous implications here for lone parenthood. The separation of marriage from motherhood is clearly important as it applies to lone parents as much as to cohabiting mothers. Lone parents are no longer quite as stigmatised as they were in the past for being unmarried or separated from a husband. It might be thought that the growing acceptability that surrounds choosing not to have children might keep the numbers of lone parents low but 'child-freedom' appears to be a choice made more frequently by middle class women and so it seems to be an important factor in the concentration of lone parenthood among the poor (see our own analysis of the FWLS in Table 1.1, Chapter 1). The relationship between motherhood and work is certainly a key issue in debates around lone motherhood. Indeed, policies to encourage lone mothers to get paid jobs could shape views more generally about working mothers.

Ideas about fatherhood, alongside ideas about masculinity, are also changing (Burgess and Ruxton 1996, Burghes *et al.* 1997). In the past, fatherhood has been equated with breadwinning. The role of a father was to provide income for his family. Fatherhood was also linked to discipline within the home rather than with caring for the child. Until the 1970s, fathers were discouraged from attending the birth of their children and the concept of a 'house-husband' – a man who voluntarily chose to stay at home and look after his children – barely existed until late on in the twentieth century. Today, fathers are expected not only to provide an income but also to participate in playing with their children and taking care of their physical and emotional needs. Fathers are expected to attend the birth of their children and some men are choosing to be the main childcarers in the family.

It is surprising, perhaps, that men are increasingly expected to play a greater caring role in the family at a time when the growth of lone parenthood has created between two and five million non-resident fathers (Bradshaw *et al.* 1999). Some of these have little, if any, contact with their children. Many pay nothing towards the costs of child-rearing. At a time when more is expected of men, more and more men are increasingly divorced (or divorcing themselves) from their children. Of course, some non-resident fathers play a major role in their children's lives and some resident fathers play a minimal role. This raises a key question about the reasons for such stark differences in the behaviour of fathers towards their children.

Ideologies about childhood and children are also changing (Qvortrup *et al.* 1994, Brannen and O'Brien 1995, 1996). The sociology of childhood has emerged since the 1970s to challenge many of the assumptions made about children in contemporary Western society (Corsaro 1997). Prior to the 1970s, children were marginalised from sociology, perhaps mainly because of their lack of power to influence the focus of debate. In social policy, children are sometimes the focus of the debate – for example in looking at child poverty or care services – but concern for children usually revolves around concern for the adults that the children will become rather than the children in their own right. In carrying out research into 'the family' many researchers have ignored the voices of children. As Hill and Tisdall state (1997: p. 74) 'systematic accounts of children's views are rare.' Now, however, an increasing body of research with children is emerging (see Daniel and Ivatts 1998). This research includes asking children about their experiences of parental separation, living on low incomes, and in lone parent families (Harrison 1996, Middleton *et al.* 1994, Clarke *et al.* 1996).

Today, children are increasingly coming to be seen as autonomous. Their testimony in court is taken more seriously than before and, if their parents separate, their views about which parent they will live with are considered important. The idea of children being able to divorce their parents is also becoming reality (Houghton-James 1994).

3.4 Defining lone parenthood

So far in this book, we have used the term 'lone parent' with minimal discussion of its definition. Lone parenthood is frequently discussed in the media or elsewhere and the term may seem fairly clear. But, as we mentioned in Chapter 1, and as has been argued elsewhere (Crow and Hardey 1992), the boundaries around lone parenthood are vague.

The boundaries around lone parenthood

Lone parents are generally defined as people who are not living with a partner but are living with dependent children. This raises two main definitional questions: how do we define 'living with a partner'? And how do we define a child as being 'dependent'?

Living with a partner

In the past, analysis of lone parenthood relied on marital status to define lone parents. It was assumed that married women with children would be living with their husband while unmarried women or widows with children would be living without a partner. But with the rise of divorce and cohabitation, such definitions became questioned and living arrangements rather than marital status became more important. There is still an issue, however, about whether cohabiting couples should be equated with married couples since cohabitation can take a variety of forms and may mean very different things to the couple.

The rise in cohabitation has meant that we need to define what is meant by 'living together'. A number of official guidelines have been developed to determine whether or not two people are cohabiting. According to the guidelines used by the Department of Social Security (see Child Poverty Action Group 1999/2000: 2/113–121), cohabitation involves members of the opposite sex who share the same household and may be in a stable relationship (Box 3.2). They may also have joint financial arrangements or share responsibilities for childcare. The couple may be having a sexual relationship and if a man and woman are publicly acknowledged to be 'a couple' this is likely to be taken as an indication that they are taking on the conventions of marriage. No single factor in the guidelines

---

Box 3.2   Indicators of cohabitation according to the Department of Social Security

- Members of the opposite sex.
- Living in the same household.
- Joint arrangements for the storage, cooking and eating of food.
- Stable relationship.
- Joint financial arrangements.
- Sharing responsibility for children.
- Sexual relationship.
- Publicly acknowledged as a couple.

Source: Child Poverty Action Group 1999/2000: 2/113–121

---

can be taken as conclusive proof that cohabitation is taking place (although it is impossible for a homosexual couple to be defined as a couple for benefit purposes even if they fulfil all other criteria). Each criterion is weighed before a final decision is reached. Similarly, the fact that a couple does not fulfil any of these criteria does not prove that they are not cohabiting. These are the official guidelines for the purposes of social security. Other official guidelines may differ; for example, some may recognise that two people of the same sex could be living as a couple.

A number of factors are therefore taken into account and, at the margins, it may not be clear whether two people are cohabiting or not. Perhaps two people have a fairly casual relationship: they maintain separate homes but stay over with each other for half of the week; they keep separate financial arrangements mostly but also share some bills. The DSS might take one view of this relationship which could be different from the view taken by the individuals involved. The people in 'the couple' may not see themselves as living with each other even though they do not dispute the objective facts about the nature of their relationship. And perhaps one member of 'the couple' feels that they are 'living with' the other person but the other does not!

One of the difficulties is that people's living arrangements and relationships have become more diverse and therefore more difficult to fit neatly into one of two simple categories (either living together or not living together). We might therefore produce the following typology to cover the

Table 3.1 Typology of couple/single living arrangements

	Living arrangements	Identity	Example(s)
1. Living with a partner	Two people live in same home	See themselves as 'a couple'	Married couple living in same home
2. Living apart, identity together	Two people living apart some of the time	See themselves as part of a couple	One partner in navy or oil rig worker, dual career couple working in different regions
3. Living together, identity apart	Two people living in the same home	Do not see themselves as part of a couple	Couple who separate emotionally but remain in same home for reasons of convenience or for sake of children
4. Living together and apart	Two people with own homes but often stay in other's home	See relationship as important but do not see themselves fully as a couple	Two people who stay over with each other for some nights of the week but retain independence in many ways, e.g. finances
5. Living without a partner	One person living in own home	No partner or may have a casual boy/girlfriend but not seen as part of a couple	Single person living on own

variety of possible arrangements as shown in Table 3.1. This typology con-centrates on two main variables: living arrangements and identity. Other variables such as financial arrangements will also be important but would probably stem from these rather than being a central factor. This typology creates five groups but, as with most typologies, it cannot capture the full complexity of people's lives and people may not fit straightforwardly in one group or another. Nevertheless it is probably a better way of classify-ing people than the simple 'living together/living alone' classification. Lone parenthood is most often associated with group 5 (living without a partner) and would not appear in group 1 (living with a partner) but could lone parents be included in groups 2 to 4?

While the DSS tries to use a judgement based mostly on objective facts to define status, most survey data on lone parenthood are now based on asking someone to define for themselves whether or not they are living with a partner. Subjective identification is therefore the basis for evidence from survey data. If someone who is living with a dependent child says that they are not living with a partner, then they will be categorised as a lone parent. They may say, moreover, that they are not living with a partner even if, by some of the more objective criteria shown above, they would be classified as doing so. The growth in lone parenthood, as reflected in survey figures, could therefore be partly a result of people increasingly defining themselves as living without a partner even though, on more objective criteria, they may appear to have a partner.

Living with a dependent child

The very concept of 'parent' is hotly contested. As we shall see in Chapter 8, it involves three main aspects: biological, social and legal. In the nineteenth century, the legal aspect was paramount. With no way of proving paternity, marriage became the only way of conferring parenthood. Towards the end of the twentieth century blood tests and then genetic tests transferred the idea of parenting from a legal phenomenon to a biological one. And in the field of child maintenance, biological parenthood is certainly the key to financial liability rather than legal or social parenthood. However, the reliance on biological parenthood becomes problematic in a world where surrogacy, IVF, egg or embryo donation are all on the increase. And the possibility of cloning takes the argument one step further. With the increase in numbers of step-parents, the notion of social parenting has gained currency. And this is certainly how children themselves view parenthood. Research with children has shown that they do not equate biology or even contact with (good) parenting (James 1999). They see the quality of the relationship in terms of feeling loved and valued as central. The opportunity to be reciprocal in the relationship by returning love and care is also considered part of the parent–child relationship.

The definition of 'living with a dependent child' may seem unproblematic at first but there are a number of difficulties with it. For example, if a couple split up and both have access to the child, do both parents become lone parents? Or is residence with a child more important than access? And if custody or care is shared, are both parents living with their child? Living with a child (or a partner) involves the concept of a household. According to family law, a household is not a physical object, like a house, but something abstract. Thus two people might live under the same roof but not live in the same household if, for example, they eat separately and do not socialise together.

Other questions revolve around issues such as: at what age do children stop being dependent? Are we talking about financial dependence only or other types, such as emotional dependence? The Child Support Agency rules reflect the complexity of defining 'dependent' children, and the Child Support Act distinguishes between 'parents with care' and 'persons with care'. A person with care has day-to-day care of a child, which must involve a minimum of two nights a week on average. A person with care need not be a person! It could be a children's home. Foster parents would also count as persons with care rather than parents. A parent includes biological parents, parents by adoption, parents by virtue of a parental order (for example following a surrogate pregnancy). Thus there are a number of aspects to parenthood.

Blurred boundaries

The difficulties in defining lone parenthood are, perhaps, most acute at the beginning and the end of a period as a lone parent. For example, if a man leaves his wife and children, does the wife immediately become a lone parent? If he returns the next day, the woman may not consider herself to have experienced lone parenthood. Then again, if she did not know whether he would return or not, she may have begun to consider her options and begun to see herself in a new way. Equally, there are difficulties defining the end of lone parenthood. If a lone parent has a boyfriend who stays over with her some nights, at what point do they become a couple? The individuals involved may view this differently from other people or other agencies, such as the Benefits Agency.

It is worth pointing out that becoming part of a couple is only one way of leaving lone parenthood. Children grow up and are no longer dependent or they might leave the lone parent's home (perhaps to live with the absent parent). If the lone parent (or an only child) dies, this family type ceases to exist.

Different types of lone parent

As we saw in Chapter 1, lone parents are often divided according to the way they became lone parents, such as:

- through the death of a spouse (widows/widowers);
- through separation or divorce from a partner; and
- through giving birth to a baby while not living with a partner.

A number of official reports separate lone parents neatly into one of these groups but, as has been argued above in relation to the general category of lone parent, the boundaries between different types of lone parent are also blurred. For example, in a qualitative study, 44 lone parents were interviewed in depth (Rowlingson and McKay 1998). Half were chosen because they had become lone parents through separation from a partner (*separated lone parents*) and half were chosen because they had become lone parents through having a baby while single (*single lone parents*). In this classification, separated lone parents included women who had separated from a cohabiting partner as well as women who had separated (and, in some cases, divorced) from a husband.

This distinction between separated and single lone mothers may seem fairly clear but in some cases it was not easy to decide which of these categories a lone mother should be placed into. For example, among the 22 *single* lone parents, 16 had never lived with a man – 8 of these had only had casual boyfriends, the other 8 had had more regular boyfriends. A further six of the 22 single lone parents had previously lived with a partner at some point in their lives. Three of these had been living with the father of their child at the time they conceived but then split up before the child was born and so were technically 'single' lone mothers (by our definition) because they had a baby while not living with a partner. Table 3.2 shows the different types of single mother who took part in the in-depth interviews.

Among the 22 *separated* lone mothers, there were also differences depending on the nature of the relationships they had been in. Most (16) had been married to the partner from whom they had separated. The remaining six had been living with someone before separating and becoming a lone parent (see Table 3.3). In some of these cases, the relationships had been fairly brief and casual and so these women may have had more in common with some of the single lone mothers than some of the women who had been married many years and then separated. Perhaps length of relationship is a more important factor than its legal status.

Table 3.2 Types of single mothers interviewed in study by Rowlingson and McKay (1998)

22 single lone mothers			
16 had never cohabited		6 had cohabited at some point previous to having their baby	
8 had casual or no boyfriends	8 had regular boyfriends	3 stopped cohabiting before conceiving	3 separated while pregnant

Table 3.3 Types of separated lone mothers interviewed in study by Rowlingson and McKay (1998)

22 separated lone mothers		
16 had separated/divorced from a marriage	3 had separated from a long-term cohabitation	3 had separated from a short-term cohabitation

In some ways, the single women who had had regular boyfriends or had separated from a cohabitation *before* the birth of a child were more similar to those who had separated from a cohabitation *after* the birth, than they were to other single mothers.

So far in this section we have emphasised the diversity in relationships. This diversity makes it difficult to classify people into discrete groups. Having said this, some women did fit into what might be called 'core' models of single and separated lone parenthood. For example, some single women had been in very casual relationships when they conceived their first child, including one woman who described her relationship with the father of her child:

> I'd known him for a while but not very well, just sort of literally to talk to in the pub.

Equally, among the women who had separated from husbands, there were what might be thought of as typical stories of women who married, then had children and then, in some cases many years later, divorced.

We might therefore split these lone mothers into four groups as in Table 3.4. At either end we have our 'core' lone mothers – those who were clearly single lone mothers and those who were clearly separated or divorced from a husband. Then there are the quasi-singles were who were

Table 3.4 Alternative typology of lone mothers

'Core' single lone mothers	Quasi-singles	Quasi-separated	'Core' separated/divorced
No regular boyfriend	Not cohabiting but had regular boyfriend	Cohabited prior to first birth or separated from a cohabitation	Separated/divorced from a marriage
8	8	12	16

Source: Rowlingson and McKay (1998)

not cohabiting but had a regular boyfriend. Finally, there were those who were quasi-separated, having cohabited before the birth of their first baby or had separated from a cohabiting partner after the birth.

3.5 Summary

While there is a great deal of sociological theory relating to the family in general, relatively few theoreticians have applied themselves specifically to analysing lone parenthood. Functionalist theories see the nuclear family as one of the essential building blocks of society and lone parenthood would be viewed, within this framework, as a dysfunctional family structure. Marxist theory traditionally ignored the family since it concentrated on the world of paid work. The family was seen as a side issue and the unpaid work carried out by women in the home was ignored. Marxist feminists have applied Marxism to issues of gender and work and other feminists have placed gender at the centre of analysis for a range of issues, including family life. Some feminists view lone parenthood as a challenge to private patriarchy (the domination of women by men in the home). But the dependence of lone parents on the state might be seen as a form of public patriarchy.

Post-modernist theories stress the diversity of human experience and the differences between individuals. Post-modernist approaches also focus on meaning, power and language. Within this framework 'discourse analysis' has been applied to lone parenthood, with a number of different discourses being identified, from 'social threat' to 'lifestyle choice' and so on. Post-modernist approaches have also encouraged more sophisticated analyses of 'groups' such as lone parents and more complex analyses of power.

It has become widely accepted that lone parenthood should be understood from a gender perspective. Thus it is argued that lone parents are poor because they are women. This is largely due to women's general disadvantage in relation to the labour market and the social security system. We argue that gender is clearly an important factor in relation to lone parenthood but that other factors, most particularly social class, are also important. Thus poverty causes lone parenthood as well as being a result of it.

With increasing diversity in the way people live their lives, it is becoming very difficult to categorise family structures. At the extremes, it may be clear when two people are living together and when one person is living on their own. But between these two extremes a variety of arrangements can occur. Similarly it is not always clear when 'a dependant' is living with a particular person. Is a child dependent on two lone parents if the parents have shared care? At what age do children cease to be 'dependent'?

Children's rights became a key theme in the 1990s. Rather than being seen as the property of their parents, children came to be seen as having rights of their own. In the past, children were expected to be 'seen but not heard' and to a large extent this was reflected in research – very few studies involved talking directly to children. This is changing now with more child-centred research studies being conducted. And the power of children as consumers (the rather derogatorily labelled 'pester power') means that some children's voices are heard by parents in some circumstances.

The role of the state

Changes in family structures, relationships and norms have major implications for the relationships between the individual, the family and the state. This is very evident from the growth of lone parenthood. Most lone parents are receiving social security and are thus financially dependent on the state. Prior to the growth of lone parenthood, most women in couples were financially dependent on the male 'breadwinner' in their family or, if the man was unemployed, on the male benefit claimant. Thus the direct dependence of women on men (who may themselves be dependent on the state) has been replaced by a more direct dependence of women on the state. This is what underlies many concerns about the growth of lone parenthood (alongside concerns about the poverty of these women and their children). As we shall see in this book, lone parents separated from a partner sometimes feel more independent as lone parents than they felt while in a couple. This is because direct dependence on the state is sometimes experienced by women as less oppressive than direct dependence on a man. The state may not pay much money but at least it is regular money with few conditions attached in terms of required behaviour (though this appears to be changing in terms of requirements to consider work).

Another way of characterising the relationship between the state and the family is that states are more concerned with intervening in the family lives of working class people than middle class people. The British state is concerned about lone mothers and absent fathers because of the class background of these groups. This chapter discusses the role of the state vis-à-vis the individual and the family, especially in relation to parents caring for children. For whom and for what is the state responsible? When is it legitimate for the state to intervene in someone's 'private' life? How is 'private' life defined? Should the state promote or encourage a particular family form?

4.1 The nature of 'the state' and the regulation of 'private' behaviour

Many books use the term 'the state' as though it is a straightforward term but it is not (see Box 4.1). Vincent (1987: p. 4) makes the following point about 'the state': 'Despite its apparent solidity (try not paying your taxes or leaving the country without a passport) it is none the less difficulty to identify – an idea or cluster of concepts, values and ideas about social existence.' In this book, we use the term 'the state' in both an organisational/institutional and also a functional manner. In organisational terms, the state is a set of governmental or quasi-governmental institutions. In functional terms, the state is a set of goals and principles pursued by various institutions and groups.

Box 4.1   Defining 'the state'

The term 'the state' is often used loosely and, indeed, there is no simple, uncontested definition. Organisational definitions of 'the state' see it as a set of institutions and organisations such as central and local government departments, the courts, the police, the army and so on. Other institutions, such as the professions, are often closely linked to it. The nature of the state varies from country to country but it is not usually a unified, internally coherent body. Each part of the state has its own policies and practices, and different parts of the state may come into conflict. Even within one particular part of the state, such as central government, different departments may have conflicting approaches. What different institutions of the state have in common is that they tend to act in ways to maintain their powerful positions. This book uses the term 'the state' in a fairly general way as described here, bearing in mind that it is not a single body with unity of purpose or outlook.

A more functional definition of the state would focus on the state's goals. The primary goal of a state has traditionally been defending the nation against other nation states and maintaining law and order within its own borders. In the twentieth century, states in the developed world have concerned themselves with the general social and economic welfare of their citizens – thus turning themselves into 'welfare states'.

The classic liberal approach to the state is to see it as an umpire between conflicting interests, such as class interests, gender interests and so on. A Marxian approach would see the state not as an umpire but as an arm of the dominant economic class. A radical feminist approach might see the state as an arm of patriarchal power. We take a pragmatic approach in this book, and see the state as both composed of, and representing, a number of vested interests. Both capitalist and patriarchal interests are among the more powerful vested interests, though the extent to which they dictate the policy and practice of the state varies over time. The election of a Labour government in 1997, for example, changed the balance of power between competing groups.

Gender, class and state

One of the main ways in which states have been classified is through a Marxian perspective. This perspective classifies states depending on their economic 'mode of production'. In very simple terms this means that some states could be defined as 'capitalist' if they involve the proletariat in selling their labour to capitalists. There have been many revisions of the Marxist approach to take into account social and economic development over time but most commentators would generally still define Western states as 'capitalist', meaning that the free market operates (although with varying degrees of freedom depending on the particular country concerned). The USA is perhaps at one extreme of the liberal-capitalist scale with continental Europe having more regulated labour and capital markets. The British state comes somewhere in between these. Class and income inequality are inherent features of capitalist countries though, once again, the degree of inequality varies.

Some feminist theorists argue that the state should primarily be seen as an instrument of patriarchy but there is great disagreement about the nature (and very existence) of patriarchy (Rowbotham 1981). One view is that it is a system allowing older men (fathers) to gain and retain power over women in particular, and to some extent, younger men (Barrett 1980). Others see it as a more general system by which men have power over women. Walby (1986: p. 51) defines patriarchy as 'a system of interrelated social structures through which men exploit women'. The institutions of state are seen, by some, as representative of patriarchal interests that subordinate women. Thus gender is the main axis of inequality in such states.

Walby (1986: p. 50) is a proponent of a 'dual systems' approach to the state. She argues that: 'patriarchy is never the only mode of production in a society but always exists in interaction with another, such as capitalism.' She argues that this can be seen in the regulation of marriage and divorce and limitations on women's rights (such as the criminalisation of abortion at certain times). Eisenstein (1979) takes a similar approach, arguing that capitalism needs patriarchy to survive, and vice versa.

Marxist and radical feminist approaches to the state are generally structuralist approaches, locating power within particular groups. Post-structuralist and/or post-modern approaches challenge the structuralist perspective. These new approaches emphasise the shifting, fragmented and complex nature of meaning and power – in fact the very notion of 'the state' would be contested within this framework (see Bauman 1992). Within this approach, power is seen as relational rather than structural, something that is exercised rather than held. Importance is placed on language and knowledge and (as we saw in Chapter 3) the power of discourse to affect the way people think and behave. These approaches offer interesting new perspectives and are valuable in challenging the fixity and status of established concepts such as class, gender and 'race'. We, however, would argue that structures of class and gender are still centrally important in the lives of lone parents, as they are in the lives of other social groups. Diversity and complexity abound in modern life but class and gender divisions remain. It is these that we focus on in relation to the role of the state.

Regulating 'private' behaviour

Theories of the state stress that its main role has traditionally been to maintain law and order. So why would it be seen as legitimate for the state to intervene in 'private' life? And how does it do this? Some behaviour is generally considered 'private' and is seen as purely the business of the individual who is engaged in that behaviour. For example, sexual behaviour is particularly likely to be seen as part of someone's 'private' life. But the state regulates sexual behaviour in a number of ways (see Evans 1993). For example, there are laws about the age of consent. In Britain, the age of consent for heterosexuals is 16. For gay men it is 18 although there have recently been strong moves to equalise this to the same age as for heterosexuals. Until 1968 it was illegal for gay men to have sex at all, at any age. Why does the state make laws in relation to sexual consent? One explanation relates to the desire to 'protect' younger people who may not be seen as having sufficient maturity to behave in their best interests before certain ages. This is a paternalistic approach. Another explanation is that the state is securing the rights of fathers over daughters until certain ages. This is a more patriarchal approach and one that does not explain why there are laws covering homosexual sex.

The law also currently prohibits certain activities even between consenting adults. For example, while it is currently legal for heterosexuals and lesbians to have group sex in private, it is currently illegal in the UK for more than two gay men to have sex with each other in private. The European Court of Human Rights has recently ruled that such prosecutions violate the right to privacy (*Guardian*, 1 August 2000) and it is likely that the UK government will abolish the relevant gross indecency laws. But the example demonstrates that the state does sometimes intervene in the most private of all activities, even those between consenting adults.

Legislation on sexual matters is one way in which the state can exercise its power. It can also exercise power by promoting the legitimacy or illegitimacy of certain types of behaviour. For example, in the 1980s, there was a backlash against the 'permissive' values apparently prevalent at the time. This backlash came to the fore when the HIV/AIDS issue first came to public attention. According to Durham (1991: p. 127), right wing Christian groups argued that the main barrier against all sexually transmitted diseases was 'sexual chastity before marriage and monogamous exclusive faithfulness after'. These groups wanted the Conservative government to take a lead in promoting appropriate behaviour. But while the Conservative government was certainly in sympathy with the view that sex was best contained within marriage, it nevertheless promoted the 'safer sex' message. The main message here was that condoms, rather than marriage and monogamy, were the best barriers against sexually transmitted diseases. In this case, a right wing government passed up the opportunity to preach morality and, instead, took a more pragmatic approach.

As well as intervening in sexual matters, the state also intervenes in other areas of 'private' life such as:

- the status of illegitimate children;
- reproductive technology and rights;
- abortion;
- adoption;
- childcare;
- the relationships between parents and children;
- marriage, divorce and cohabitation.

This chapter highlights two areas for further discussion of the role of the state in relation to family life: the right to reproduce and children's rights.

4.2 The right to reproduce: direct and indirect state intervention

The state plays a key role in reproduction. It is currently illegal for certain groups of people to have sex (e.g. under-age people), to marry (e.g. siblings), or to be helped to have children (e.g. those in closed prisons are denied 'the right' to conceive children with their partners). For some women with learning disabilities sterilisation has been sought.

The growth of the family planning movement in the early part of the twentieth century is a fascinating story. The movement was partly inspired by the desire to give women greater control of their reproduction so that they could regulate the number and timing of any children they might have. But it was also inspired by ideas from eugenics that promoted the aim of genetically engineering a more 'healthy' race of people. These ideas usually involved 'purifying' 'the race' of undesirable groups, including parts of the working class. As Searle (1976: p. 113) points out: 'the pioneers of eugenics in Britain, almost without exception, were from comfortable middle class backgrounds and class prejudice all too often crept into their evaluation of their scientific work.' Many eugenicists thought that IQ tests could be used to identify objectively those people whose reproduction should be encouraged and those people whose reproduction should be discouraged or even prevented. They did not realise that these IQ tests were heavily biased in favour of the middle classes. Some eugenicists, however, were quite open about the benefits they saw from reducing those members of the working classes who were the least intelligent. They thought that: 'the elimination of the pauper and the wastrel would immensely increase the productivity of the workforce' (Searle 1976: p. 49). Taxes would be reduced as there would be fewer unproductive mouths for the tax-payer to feed. McLaren (1978) argues that the later eugenicists were afraid of the power of the working classes. Some argued that infectious diseases such as TB should not be eradicated because they were a useful way of 'weeding out' the weakest members of society. McLaren (1978: p. 215) argues that, for eugenicists 'the issue of fertility control had as its central concern the reproductive habits of the working classes.'

It might be thought that the eugenicists in Britain remained a minority group with little power. But, largely due to their lobbying, the Mental Deficiency Act was passed in 1913. It did not go as far as some eugenicists would have liked but it did legislate for the detention and institutionalisation of the 'mentally deficient' on a sex-segregated basis (to avoid any conceptions). These so-called 'defectives' included, according to Soloway (1990): certain categories of pauper; habitual drunkards; and women on poor relief giving birth to illegitimate children. Thus single lone mothers could be labelled as mentally deficient and locked away in the first half of the twentieth century. Some American states went even further. They compulsorily sterilised, sexually segregated or forbade the marriage of people with mental illness or impairment, alcohol dependency, sexually transmitted diseases and those who were considered to be both promiscuous and poor.

Eugenicists in Britain wanted the 1913 Act to be the start of a raft of legislation but, as Soloway (1990: p. 107) suggests: 'they recognized correctly that the country's long tradition of individual liberties . . . precluded any serious governmental intrusion into the most private areas of people's lives – marriage, sex and childbearing.' The state therefore moved away from legislation towards education, persuasion and incentives. And the eugenics movement became heavily tarred with the brush of Nazism as it came to be linked with Hitler's ideas of creating a master race. However, in recent years, the human genome project has revived discussions about the desirability and feasibility of genetic engineering. Should certain 'defective genes' be screened out to prevent babies being born with particular diseases? Should parents be able to choose the eye colour of their child or any other physical (or perhaps psychological) trait?

The medical world marches on and the increasing research into the human genome will no doubt keep the debate over genetic engineering high on the public and scientific agenda. Today, states directly intervene in reproduction as far as abortion, adoption and fertility treatment are concerned. States also intervene indirectly – through education and the tax and benefit systems – to discourage poor women (especially those in their teenage years) from having children. In Britain, the state is very keen to reduce the numbers of teenage pregnancies (see Chapter 1). It could be argued that such discouragement is designed to prevent greater poverty for both the women and their children. However, the state's concern to reduce tax expenditure is also a great motivator for policy, as is a desire to contain what is perceived by some to be a dangerous underclass.

In some US states, the state uses the benefit system to discourage lone parents from having further children, through 'family caps'. The Personal Responsibility and Work Opportunity Reconciliation Act of 1996 was a compromise between the Democrat agenda that aimed to help lone parents into employment and the Republican agenda 'to end illegitimacy and family break-up'. The Act attempted to meet these two aims 'by eliminating aid to teen mothers, barring aid for additional children and children without paternity established, and imposing time limits on assistance even if a woman was working' (Waldfogel 1997). The Democrat agenda was 'to end welfare as we know it' whereas the Republican agenda was to end the growth in numbers of lone parent families.

The 1996 Act ended the absolute entitlement status of welfare and introduced a capped block grant in the form of Temporary Assistance to Needy Families (TANF). Thus there is no guarantee that any assistance will be available for those in need (although Food Stamps and Medicaid are available to all those eligible). The Act also introduced time limits for welfare: a two-year time limit for a woman receiving TANF unless she was working; and a five-year lifetime limit even if a woman was working. The states, however, are allowed to exempt up to 20 per cent from these rules if they have good cause. Time limits gained widespread support among the American public but Waldfogel (1997) points out that these limits will have a devastating effect on the women and children in lone parent families. States are permitted to impose a family cap (a ban on additional benefits for new children born on welfare) although research suggests that such policies have little impact on the birth rate (Sawhill 1995).

So the USA has gone a long way both to encourage poor lone parents into employment and to discourage women from becoming lone parents. In relation to this, Jencks and Edin (1995) have posed the challenging question 'Do poor women have the right to bear children?' They argue that many social policies are based on the premise that:

> people should not have children until they are ready to support them. Yet for many poor women, that time will never come. Sad to say, there are neither enough good jobs nor enough good husbands to provide every American woman with enough money to support a family. Are we to assume that the losers in this lottery have no right to bear children at all? And if not, are we really prepared to enforce this principle and all of its implications? (p. 43)

It is clear that there are different ways in which the state can intervene in reproduction. It can directly legislate to ban or permit certain types of activity. Or it can introduce policies that indirectly encourage or discourage certain types of activity.

4.3 Children's rights

The way in which parents deal with their children has hitherto been seen as beyond the legitimate scope of state intervention. In the past, children were seen as the property of their fathers and the state kept well away from interfering with father's rights. However, the movement in favour of increased children's rights has legitimised increased state intervention, with the state portraying itself as the protector of children's rights.

In the past, the nature of obligations between parents and children received relatively little attention in law. Where they were addressed, marriage was seen as a sufficient basis for creating a legal relationship between parent and child. In the classic legal text by Blackstone (1775), two sorts of children are distinguished: 'legitimate, and spurious, or bastards'. Blackstone argues that a parent's obligations to a legitimate child involve maintenance, protection and education. In practice, it was not the parents but more specifically the father of a legitimate child that had obligations and rights over that child. Turning to illegitimate children, parents had few obligations or rights in law towards children born out of wedlock. Such children had no legally recognised guardians and neither mother nor father had any 'right' to custody. However, Blackstone did argue that there was one area that parents of illegitimate children should be responsible for – child support: 'although bastards are not looked upon as children to any civil purposes, yet the ties of nature, of which maintenance is one, are not so easily dissolved.' If the ties of nature were insufficiently strong to ensure adequate child support then Justices of the Peace had powers to enforce parents of illegitimate children to support them financially. So parents of illegitimate children had no legal rights or responsibilities towards these children except in the field of child support. It seems that the concerns of tax-payers dictated views of what parental obligations were enshrined in law.

The old Poor Law had placed a general obligation on parents to support their children. But in 1844, the Poor Law Amendment Act permitted an unmarried mother to obtain a magistrates' court order against the father requiring him to support both herself and her illegitimate child. This was the first occasion on which any father had acquired a direct support duty towards his child (Maclean and Eekelaar 1997). Later statutes extended the provisions to married women (although the divorce courts had always been able to make child support provisions).

By the end of the nineteenth century, mothers of *illegitimate* children were, in practice, gaining recognition of broader responsibilities and rights but mothers still had relatively few rights over *legitimate* children. It was as late as 1973 when mothers obtained the same rights as fathers over their legitimate children and in 1987 the Family Law Reform Act made further changes in this field. This act removed many of the remaining distinctions in law between children born inside and outside of wedlock. However, some still remain, such as the distinction between a father's legal relationship with a child born outside marriage and a father's legal relationship with a child born inside marriage (see Chapter 7).

The Children Act 1989 created the concept of 'parental responsibility' and enacted that, while married parents automatically would have parental responsibility over their children, in the case of children born outside marriage only the mother would have automatic parental responsibility. The child's father has to apply for it either with the agreement of the mother or with a court order. This does not mean that unmarried fathers have no rights or responsibilities at all. In practice, they tend to exercise many of the usual rights and responsibilities of fatherhood, particularly if they are living with the mother but if separated from the mother, these come into question. And even if they live with the mother, their rights and responsibilities can be challenged. For example, a doctor could quite safely accept an unmarried father's consent for medical treatment for their child but they could also, quite legitimately, refuse to accept such authorisation.

In the 1980s, the Gillick case brought the issue of parental responsibility to the fore. Victoria Gillick took her local health authority to court because it advised doctors that they could lawfully offer young people under 16 confidential advice about contraception. Gillick felt that, as a parent, she had the right to be informed by the GP if a child of hers sought advice about contraception. After a long legal battle, the House of Lords eventually ruled that 'parental right yields to the child's right to make his own decisions when he reaches a sufficient understanding and intelligence to be capable of making up his mind on the matter requiring decision' (quoted in Rogers and Roche 1994: p. 218). This ruling leaves great discretion (and therefore power) to GPs, and ultimately the courts, to decide when particular children pass this test.

The Children Act 1989 is the most important recent reform in this field. Parton (1991: p. 1) argues that this Act was 'an attempt to address some of the most sensitive and potentially explosive issues concerning the relationship between the child, the family and various state agents'. The Act introduced a new balance between the need to protect children and the need to enable parents to challenge state intervention. Before the Act, a liberal state such as Britain had always faced a dilemma in terms of the amount and nature of state intervention in the family. State intervention was usually seen as a last resort unless children were at risk of very serious harm from other members of their family. In the 1980s, a number of well-publicised cases had demonstrated that prevailing arrangements were failing.

The deaths of a number of children, particularly Jasmine Beckford (in 1985), Kimberley Carlile and Tyra Henry (both in 1987) showed that the state had failed to protect these children from abuse within the family. Social workers had intervened too little and too late to protect these children. They had shown too much concern for parental rights and the privacy of 'the family'. But on the other hand, in the Cleveland affair in 1987 some agents of the state (doctors and social workers) were removing children from families with only dubious medical indications of abuse. In this case, professionals had failed to recognise the rights and autonomy of parents and children by intervening too soon and too heavy-handedly. Changes were therefore needed in the law and also in the practices and attitudes of a range of professionals, particularly social workers and health professionals.

The Children Act 1989 made social workers more accountable for their actions and made courts the explicit focus for adjudication where parental powers and responsibilities were transferred to the state. Parton (1991) outlines the major principles of the Act including the following:

1. The upbringing of children is seen as primarily the responsibility of parents. The state will only intervene to help out in cases of need.

2. Services to families in need should be arranged in voluntary partnership with parents. The emphasis should be on maintaining family relationships and contact as much as possible.

3. Parents' legal powers and responsibilities for a child should only be transferred to the state (a local authority in this case) following a full court hearing. The court should be satisfied that there is evidence of significant harm or the likelihood of such harm

4. In such cases, the interests of the child are paramount but parents should be properly represented

Parton (1991: p. 155) concludes that 'the role of the state was confirmed as residual and supportive rather than primary.' The family was seen as a private institution but parents were now seen as having responsibilities towards their children rather than holding parental property rights as they had effectively done in the past.

Even with the Children Act in place, parents have quite far-reaching rights over their children. For example, it is quite legal for parents in Britain to subject their children to 'reasonable chastisement'. Wheen (2000) argues that this legal right explains a recent case where a man was acquitted of actual bodily harm even though he had regularly beaten his small stepson with a three-foot (one-metre) cane, causing prolonged bruising. The European Court of Human Rights subsequently ruled, in September 1998, that British law had failed to protect the boy from 'cruel and degrading punishment' and that the government should do something about it. Eight countries in Europe have already banned all physical punishment of children (including by parents), with Sweden leading the way in 1979. But the British government appears to have no intention of banning such punishment. It has merely produced a consultation document explaining what 'reasonable chastisement' means. Much of the argument about physical punishment of children echoes that of physical punishment of women by their husbands in a previous era. Wheen (2000) quotes from the eighteenth century jurist, William Blackstone, who argued that 'As he is to answer for her misbehaviour the law thought it reasonable to entrust him with that power of restraining her, by domestic chastisement, in the same moderation that a man is allowed to correct his apprentices or children.'

The law no longer permits men to physically punish their wives although it is only relatively recently that the police, the courts and the public have taken domestic violence seriously. As in most 'family matters' some people do not think it appropriate to 'interfere' between parents and children unless serious harm is being caused.

The issue of Children's Rights has gained greater attention in recent years and in 1991 the UK government ratified the UN Convention on the Rights of the Child. But this convention is not enforceable in the British courts of law and it is unlikely that children's rights will be given equal weight as women's rights given the continuing powerlessness of this group. The state in Britain enforces a very negative version of children's rights – it aims to prevent children from being seriously harmed by others but it does little to promote a positive level of quality of life for children. In relation to lone parenthood there is much more concern with securing child support than in ensuring that absent parents play a positive role in their child's lives (in terms of contact and care).

4.4 Approaches to family policy

So far in this chapter we have seen that there are different ways in which the state might intervene in family life. Such intervention has been categorised in a number of different ways. For example, Fox Harding (1996) categorises family policy on a continuum from the authoritarian to the liberal. Authoritarian approaches attempt to enforce 'certain preferred behaviour patterns and family forms' and prohibit others (Fox Harding 1996: p. 179). Such an approach could only be successful in an authoritarian state where personal freedom is severely limited. An extreme example of this is the Chinese government's regulations on the number of children that can be born within a family. The aim of this policy is to contain the population. In Romania after the Second World War, however, an equally authoritarian regime attempted to force the population to expand itself, for example, by banning abortion. Authoritarian approaches are likely to be accompanied by certain ideologies of the family and these would be presented through the mechanism of propaganda. Such states might also seek to engineer particular attitudes and cultural beliefs in such a way that people police themselves. These internal controls, however, are very difficult to maintain and so authoritarian regimes tend to rely on coercion and punishments to deter people from non-conformity to the prescribed policy. In the case of Romania tough action was taken against those suspected of having or carrying out an illegal abortion.

According to Fox Harding, liberal approaches to family policy allow people to decide for themselves exactly how they want to arrange their family life. The state has no particular family ideology and allows people to choose how to live their lives. There is therefore no explicit family policy as the state is relatively neutral and has no aims to change people's behaviour or attitudes. However, it is difficult to imagine what a 'neutral' family policy could be like. Most policies tend to affect families indirectly if not directly and some families benefit more than others from different policies. As Fox Harding (1996: p. 185) herself admits, the liberal approach 'is not neutral towards families but reinforces pre-existing patterns which may be very adverse for some groups'. Families differ and they have interests that often compete with each other. One policy might benefit a lone parent family while disadvantaging a couple family.

Between the authoritarian and liberal approaches lie a range of intermediate models of family policy. Some might try to enforce family responsibilities in particular areas (such as child support for example). Some might manipulate incentives to create and sustain particular family types (such as providing financial incentives to marry or have children). Some might seek to support families where they fail or malfunction in some respect (for example in providing residential homes for children. And some might merely respond to the needs of families as these change over time. Rather than use Fox Harding's classification as a way of classifying individual nation states, it is more helpful to use it to see how states use different approaches at different times and in different fields of family policy. Thus one state can employ enforcement in one area of family life, incentives in another, supporting families in another and responding to needs in another.

It can be argued that the British approach is eclectic, taking aspects of all the intermediate models highlighted by Fox Harding. But perhaps it comes closest to another of her intermediate models whereby the 'state's actions are based upon certain assumptions about how families operate, and these are built into policies' (Fox Harding 1996: p. 191). Thus there have traditionally been no specific policy goals relating to the family in British policy but certain assumptions such as the assumption of women's economic dependence on men have been built into policy. It is also assumed that the parent–child unit is a single, harmonious unit and that children are dependent on their parents. The consequences of these assumptions can be illustrated within the field of social security policy. Here, there is an assumption that money is shared within the family and that the man is the head of the household. Hence in couple families, most social security benefits are paid to the man on the assumption that he will then distribute it fairly to the other members of the family. These assumptions do not, however, reflect reality in all cases. Research with lone parents reveals that although they have very little income, they sometimes feel better off as lone parents because they have money paid directly to them, rather than having to rely on the discretionary power of a male partner.

Fox Harding (1996) reminds us that the relationship between the state and the family is not one way. The state can have a powerful impact on the family but the family can also have an impact on the state, for example by voting for a particular party with a particular view of family life. And just as the state is not a unified phenomenon, so too there are different types of families, some of which will be supported by the state and some of which will be vilified.

Rather than distinguishing between authoritarian and liberal family policies, Kamerman and Kahn (1978) have placed greater emphasis on distinguishing between explicit and implicit family policies. According to this distinction, explicit family policies are those in which 'the family' is the direct target of the policy in terms of family structure or resources. Thus any reform of Child Benefit, child support, childcare services and so on would be included within explicit family policy even though the goals of the policy might not be solely or mainly related to their effect on families. For example, the goal might be to cut government spending. Implicit policies are not aimed at changing family structures and resources but might nevertheless affect them indirectly. For example, policies relating to housing, health and education might have indirect effects on family life. Implicit family policies could cover almost any area of social policy and so the category can only be defined in terms of the goals and effects of different social policies.

Millar (1998) builds on Kamerman and Kahn (1978) but prefers the terms direct/indirect to explicit/implicit. She identifies three main areas of direct family policy:

1. The legal regulation of family behaviour for example in the fields of marriage, divorce, sexual behaviour, contraception, abortion, parental responsibility and child protection.

2. Policies to support family income. This would include benefits for families with children and child support.

3. Provision of services including child care, subsidised housing and social services.

Wasoff and Dey (2000) consider the role played by the family and focus on social policies that perform similar functions. Thus they focus on social policy in the fields of: reproduction; socialisation; care and protection; resource distribution; and work. However, the family also plays an important role in other fields such as health and education. But if these other areas are included, the scope of policy becomes very wide again.

Millar (1998) considers the issue of family policy from a different perspective by categorising the ways that policy-makers and politicians might approach family matters. She identifies three perspectives: reactionary; egalitarian; and pragmatic. The reactionary perspective seeks to implement policies that will restore, preserve and support the 'traditional' family – that is, the nuclear family. Marriage is the key institution that reactionaries wish to support through policy reform. The libertarian approach takes a more sceptical view of the 'traditional' family. It sees the traditional family as responsible for the reproduction of class and gender inequalities. It wishes to use social policies to reduce these inequalities and in the process, the breakdown of the traditional family is welcomed. The pragmatic approach seeks to accept the increasing diversity in family life and support all types of family.

Gauthier (1996) also looks at family policy from the perspective of policy-makers' goals. His categorisation is similar to that of Millar (1998) and he uses it to classify family policies in different countries. He identifies four types of approach to family policy:

1. Pro-natalist states are concerned about increasing the birth rate (as in France).

2. Pro-traditionalist states (such as Germany) devise policies to support 'traditional families'.

3.   Pro-egalitarian states aim to promote equality in family life (as in Sweden)

4.   Pro-family states (such as the USA) only intervene in family life selectively as they see the family as part of the 'private sphere'.

Kamerman and Kahn (1978) have categorised family policies in European countries in a different way: those with explicit and comprehensive family policies (such as in Sweden, Norway and France); those in which family policy is seen as a field covering various policies (such as in Austria and Denmark); and those in which family policy is implicit and reluctant (such as the USA). Where does Britain stand in relation to other countries? Until recently, Britain would have been categorised with the USA as being reluctant to intervene in family life but the election of a Labour government in 1997 changed this slightly. The Labour government appears to straddle the pro-egalitarian and pro-traditional categories, perhaps creating for itself a 'Third Way' in family policy.

4.5 UK government strategy: *Supporting Families*

In the 1950s, British policy towards the family had been framed by the post-war Welfare State settlement. Millar (1999) identifies three basic principles of this settlement: full employment; male breadwinners; and stable families. The family was seen, at this time, as a private institution, beyond the scope of government except in extreme cases. Domestic violence within the family was tolerated unless children in particular were at risk of very serious injury. In the 1960s and 1970s, the traditional family appeared to be under strain with increasing numbers of divorce and increasing numbers of women in employment. Child poverty was also identified as an important issue and the feminist movement put the private sphere firmly on the public agenda, with phrases such as 'the personal is political'. So from a number of perspectives (right wing, left wing, feminist), 'the family' was becoming a hotly debated issue. The state could no longer shy away from intervention in family matters and in 1977, the Prime Minister, James Callaghan, stated that Britain needed, for the first time, a 'national family policy'. He said that the aim of this would be 'to strengthen the stability and quality of family life in Britain.' A central concern for this policy was to enable women to remain 'at the center of the family' even if they had paid jobs (Kamerman and Kahn 1997: p. 95).

The 1979 General Election ended Britain's brief 'national family policy' spell. The Conservative government was firmly non-interventionist, particularly in relation to private matters such as family life. In some ways this non-interventionism thwarted Conservative dreams of returning to traditional family life as policies to engineer family change were frowned upon even if the goals were cherished. But while the government would not bring in direct family policies to promote traditional family forms, it did create a moral climate in which certain family types were admired and others were frowned upon. Any attempt to preach private morality (such as the 'Back to Basics' campaign under John Major), however, was generally abandoned following media revelations of 'sleazy behaviour' by politicians.

After decades of non-interventionism in family life, the election of a Labour government in 1997 signalled the start of what seemed to be a new approach. It introduced a Minister for Women, a Women's Unit (in the Cabinet Office) and a Minister for Family Policy. It also issued a consultative document *Supporting Families* declaring its views about the family (Home Office 1998) but acknowledged in the paper on page 30 that: 'governments have to be very careful in devising policies that affect our most intimate relationships.' Like the previous Conservative government, the Labour government is not immune from embarrassment in this field, with the family life of the Home Secretary, Jack Straw, and the Prime Minister, Tony Blair, coming under greatest scrutiny.

The *Supporting Families* Green Paper stated that 'it is not for the state to decide whether people marry or stay together', but it went on to declare somewhat contradictorily, 'we are therefore proposing measures to strengthen the institution of marriage.' Oddly enough, many of the measures in the paper were concerning the divorce process. The government argued that it did have a right to intervene in the family if children were involved and to some extent this demonstrates the growing importance of children's rights in relation to parental rights.

The consultative document talks of supporting families rather than lecturing them about how to behave. It tries to take a humble tone, recognising the difficulties in family life and trying to help people with them. But it steers an untenable course between arguing in favour or marriage while at the same time not criticising other family arrangements. On page 4 it states:

> children need stability and security. Many lone parents and
> unmarried couples raise their children every bit as successfully as
> married parents. But marriage is still the surest foundation for raising
> children and remains the choice of the majority of people in Britain.
> We want to strengthen the institution of marriage to help more
> marriages succeed.

The government is clearly trying to have its wedding cake and eat it. It either believes that marriage is better than other family types or that it is not. Is it stability and security it supports most or the institution of marriage? The government is holding up the ideal of the stable, happy, married couple providing stable and secure family life. It sees this as the best model and one that should be supported. In so doing it will indirectly (if not directly) discriminate against other family forms. Research discussed in Chapter 7 does not generally support the government's view that marriage is necessarily the best family structure within which to raise children but this is certainly the view that the current government takes.

The document has a whole chapter devoted to 'strengthening marriage' in which it discusses its intention to provide couples intending to marry with a clear statement of their rights and responsibilities in relation to income, property, tax and benefits, and children. It also wants to help people prepare for marriage better by giving them more time to think and be counselled before they actually take the plunge. It wishes to give more support to marriages in difficulty and to try to 'save' marriages before divorce. These policies are rather tentative and weak ways of strengthening marriage and they are being considered at a time when financial incentives to marry (such as through the tax system) have been abolished. Strangely perhaps, the chapter in the document entitled 'strengthening marriage' pays far more attention to policies about divorce than it does to policies about marriage.

In relation to family life more generally, the government has proposed the following schemes and policies:

- The setting up of a National Family and Parenting Institute to give advice to people about family and parenting matters.

- A National Parenting Helpline.

- An increased role for Health Visitors in giving advice and support.

- The Sure Start scheme – a £540 million initiative to help children and their parents in their early years.

- Better financial support for families.

- Help for families to balance work and home commitments.

Despite all these schemes, the government (Home Office 1998: p. 31) still recognises that: 'family matters are essentially private matters and individuals must live their own lives.' And nearly three years after the publication of the Consultative Document, there had been no response to the consultation, so perhaps policy-making in this area is more complex and sensitive than even this government has acknowledged. One of the problems in supporting marriage is that some marriages are highly damaging to the individuals involved. The Consultative Document acknowledges this with the shocking statistic that there were an estimated 835,000 incidents of domestic violence in 1997 according to the British Crime Survey. One woman in nine is subjected to severe beatings by her partner and children often suffer neglect and abuse in such families (see also Chapter 2).

It is difficult to classify the Labour government's new approach. It is still cautious about intervention as it equates this with social engineering and preaching to people about how to live their lives. It certainly sees marriage as an important institution in line with more reactionary/ traditional perspectives. But it also recognises that other types of families need support, thus adopting a more pragmatic line.

4.6 Summary

The growth of lone parenthood has changed the relationships between men, women and the state. The direct dependence of women on men (who might themselves be dependent on the state) has been replaced by a more direct dependence of women on the state. To some extent it seems that women find dependence on the state to be less oppressive than dependence on a man. Benefit levels are low but they are reliable. The state may require lone parents to start thinking about paid work but at least the state does not require women to have the dinner on the table at a certain time and it is not physically violent to them.

So the state allows lone parents to survive financially by paying them social security benefits. It also provides accommodation for them. The state also plays a number of other roles in relation to family life more generally. In fact, perhaps there is no part of life that is considered too private to be beyond state concern. However, the state generally stands back from intervening in family life unless children are at serious threat of harm. It seems that children's rights are relatively weak, when the best the state is prepared to do is prevent serious harm rather than ensure a positively good quality of upbringing for children. The state seeks to force non-resident parents to pay maintenance but does little even to encourage these parents to provide care and love for their children. The state is more concerned with the interests of tax-payers than the interests of children.

In the past, the British state has played a major role in regulating the right to reproduce. The eugenics movement helped bring about the 1913 Mental Deficiency Act which went so far as to detain and institutionalise certain groups including poor single mothers. The idea of forcibly sterilising the poor would horrify many today but some social policies in the USA are, in effect, amounting to something similar. For example, some states refuse to pay any more money to women who have children while claiming welfare. And states have time limits for lone parents claiming welfare, though with varying degrees of effective enforcement. Some states have introduced contraceptive implants for those claiming benefit. In effect, these states are saying that poor women should not have children and they will be financially punished if they do. The mechanism is rather different from permanent and forcible sterilisation but for women with little prospect of being able to 'afford' to have a child and be independent of the state, the outcome might be similar. This is eugenics by another name. The British state has yet to take this route but it is increasingly keen to encourage lone parents to take paid work. The option of remaining on benefit indefinitely as a lone parent is fading.

British governments have traditionally been shy of pursuing a particular 'family policy' but the Labour government elected in 1997 produced a consultative document outlining its views in this area. The fact that there has been no document following from this one suggests that the government appreciates the difficulties and dangers of making interventions in family life. The government is currently trying to walk the tightrope of promoting marriage while at the same time not denigrating other family forms. This is an impossible balancing act to maintain.

part two

Lone parent families
and social policy

Part One of this book looked at lone parent families in context. It began by reviewing the profile of lone parent families today. Chapter 1 showed us that lone parents are mostly women from working class backgrounds. A growing number are single women, some of whom have cohabited in the past, some of whom have not. Non-resident parents mirror lone parents to some extent, being mostly men from working class backgrounds. Chapter 2 showed that the rise in lone parenthood over the past three decades or so is not some new phenomenon but, to some extent, represents a return to informal patterns of family life that existed in pre-industrial Britain. Some argue that this move is a retrograde step towards the 'death of the family'. Others argue that post-industrial society is breaking free from the straightjacket of Victorian family life that dominated the industrial age.

Chapter 3 outlined some conceptual and theoretical frameworks that could be applied to lone parenthood. In this book, class and gender are the two key concepts deserving of special attention in relation to lone parenthood. This is not to argue that they are sufficient in themselves to understand the experiences of lone parents. Other factors (such as ethnicity, age, sexuality, disability and locality) are also likely to be highly important to lone parents. But gender and class are very important factors and while gender has received considerable attention in the past the role of class has received much less attention.

Chapter 4 considered the role of the state in relation to lone parent families. We argue that the state is particularly concerned with lone parent families because the state has, for some time, tried to control working class morality and family patterns. The state wields power in relation to many

chapter 5

Poverty and social security

In Britain, poverty is one of the causes of lone parenthood, as well as (in Britain) one of its most likely consequences. This is especially true in relation to single lone mothers. Lone parents and their children are among the poorest groups in Britain and there has been an association between poverty and lone parenthood throughout history (see Chapter 1). Non-resident fathers also tend to live on lower than average levels of income (see Chapter 8).

As a result of low levels of employment and low rates of receiving maintenance or other forms of income, most lone parent families in Britain today receive means-tested benefits (principally, Income Support for non-workers and Working Families Tax Credit, for workers). Even a majority of those lone parents in paid work rely on income-related assistance to top up their incomes.

This chapter begins with an outline of state support for lone parents through the social security and tax systems. It then considers the extent to which this support prevents or alleviates poverty within lone parent families. The third section discusses the debates around the underclass, dependency and social exclusion. The chapter ends with a summary of recent and current government policy in this area.

5.1 The social security system

One of the aims of the social security system is to alleviate poverty. Research quoted in Chapter 1 showed that the main safety net in the British system, Income Support, does not prevent lone parents from experiencing poverty but it does prevent them from sinking too deeply into poverty. The majority of lone parent families (52 per cent) are receiving Income Support (Marsh *et al.* 2001). This section reviews the main benefits received by lone parents and the role of 'family benefits' within the overall system.

Social security is one of the policy arenas in which the state plays a vital role in relation to lone parent families. It could be used in a number of ways, including the following:

- Means-tested benefits could be paid at a fairly minimal level, allowing lone parent families to survive on benefit but do little more than that. Lone parents could then be left to decide whether or not to take paid jobs with the state remaining relatively neutral about the mother/worker issue (and providing relatively little support whatever they decide to do).

- Benefits to top up low wages could be used to encourage lone parents to take up paid work. And lone parents on benefit could be given advice and encouragement to (re-)join the labour market. In this case the state would be taking a pro-worker stance.

- Social security benefits could be paid at generous levels to women looking after children. This would be in recognition of the importance of childcare and would prevent children in lone parent families from suffering poverty. In this case the state would be taking a pro-mother stance.

- Social security levels could be paid at generous levels to women looking after children but there could also be advice, encouragement and in-work benefits to help lone parents who wish to take on paid work. In this case the state would be neutral about the mother/worker issue but would be providing a high level of support to women whatever their decision.

The first of these strategies existed in Britain until the late 1970s when the second one began to develop alongside it. In the late 1990s/early twenty-first century, the government appears keen to raise means-tested benefit levels for jobless families with children but it would be costly to raise them to 'generous' levels and high levels might act to deter lone parents from taking paid work. The third and fourth strategies are not therefore ones that the British government is likely to develop significantly.

Mayer (1997) has divided income policies for families into four categories as follows:

1.   Type A policies mainly provide cash and non-cash transfers to improve the material well-being of poor families.

2.   Type B policies require parents and children to live in group
      quarters as a way of discouraging certain types of behaviour seen
      as responsible for their poverty.

3.   Type C policies separate parents from children in an attempt to
      break the apparent cycle of disadvantage.

4.   Type D policies provide supervision of poor parents who look
      after their children at home.

Each of these types of policies has been in operation in Britain at
different times. Type A policies include the system of poor relief in the
nineteenth century but also income support in the twenty-first century.
Type B policies include nineteenth century workhouses. Type C policies
include putting children into orphanages, care homes or up for adoption
and, until the 1970s, pressure was often put on unwed mothers to give
their babies away. Type D policies might include work requirements made
on lone parents in order to receive benefit, a policy strategy that appears
to be developing now.

Benefits received by lone parents

Social security includes the range of cash benefits that are available
to families in particular circumstances. They include such benefits as
Child Benefit, the Retirement Pension, Housing Benefit and Jobseeker's
Allowance. Figures for 2000/01 show a total of £19.2 billion spent on
families and £11.3 billion spent on lone parents (Department of Social
Security 2000a). This is a very large amount of money but it should be
put in the context of a total social security budget of about £100 billion.
Thus spending on lone parents accounts for only 10 per cent of the overall budget. The reason for concern about this component of the benefits
bill is that, over the last 30 years, it has been rising as a proportion of the
overall budget. Concerns also revolve around the nature of the claimant
group – are lone parents 'deserving' of state assistance? Do they deliberately become lone parents to get social security? Should the state be
supporting a lone parent family rather than both biological parents?

Lone parents receive the same types of benefit as other parents,
namely: Child Benefit, Income Support, Housing Benefit and Working
Families Tax Credit. Benefits for widows are a relatively small part of the
overall system but, as we shall see, insurance against widowhood was
one of the first social security provisions enacted early this century.

It is customary to divide benefits into three main types (McKay and
Rowlingson, 1999: Chapter 1). First, so-called contributory benefits or

social insurance. These are benefits provided to people in particular circumstances, who can meet a test of having made enough insurance contributions (National Insurance in the UK) while in paid work. In most countries, these types of benefits tend to be relatively generous, and to enjoy popular support. Second, there are means-tested benefits. These are paid to people in certain circumstances, who have less than a specified amount of income from various sources. In some countries, and at some times, these have been perceived as being stigmatising, perhaps because they do not appear to depend on having made some kind of prior contribution to qualify. Third, there are categorical or contingent benefits, paid without any test of contribution or means to those with particular needs. The State Retirement Pension is contributory; Housing Benefit is means-tested; Child Benefit is categorical.

As far as lone parents are concerned, the social security system provides insurance against widowhood but there are currently no benefits in the UK providing insurance against separation or divorce. On divorce, an ex-wife is not entitled to any of her ex-husband's credits for unemployment assistance or incapacity benefit. However, new rules were introduced from December 2000 following the Welfare Reform and Pensions Act 1999 to cover pension splitting on divorce. These split any pension rights into two separate rights at the time of divorce.

Only one lone mother in ten is a widow, and the proportion has been falling over time. The others may be eligible for general National Insurance or means-tested benefits. But because they are women, and more specifically mothers, the earnings records of most lone mothers means that they are not entitled to National Insurance benefits. According to Marsh et al. (2001) only 1 per cent of lone parents were receiving Jobseeker's Allowance in 1999 and 3 per cent Incapacity Benefit (the two main insurance benefits for working-age people).

Hence most of those who receive benefits are on means-tested benefits. These are set at a minimum level and evidence shows that lone mothers have a very low standard of living, sometimes for very long periods. The majority of lone parents (52 per cent) receive Income Support. This figure increases to 68 per cent for single lone mothers. Income Support is the basic safety net benefit. It provides just enough to allow people to survive on and yet more than half of all families on this benefit are having money deducted from this basic amount of money, primarily to repay funds from the social fund (Marsh et al. 2001). This, clearly, leaves them with even less to survive on.

Numerous independent academic studies have been carried out into benefit levels and they all show that these levels are woefully inadequate to allow people to participate in society in any meaningful way (Veit-Wilson 1999). A number of studies have found that social assistance (Income Support) levels are only between two-thirds and three-quarters of the level required for 'minimal participation' in society or 'minimal adequacy' (Townsend 1979, Mack and Lansley 1985, Oldfield and Yu 1993).

Qualitative research with lone mothers has asked them about how and why they became lone mothers and what life is like as a lone parent (Rowlingson and McKay 1998). One lone mother interviewed for this study spoke for many when she explained that life on benefit is:

> . . . impossible. Every month there are three or four bills that you are
> not going to be able to pay. I spend my whole time on the phone
> saying, 'I'll pay you that next month' or 'I'll pay half of that' . . . and
> leaving things until it gets to the point where – not quite to the
> point of bailiffs – but you're just buying time all the time . . . You
> have never got enough money, ever. There's never a week goes by
> where I am sitting at the end of a week and there's £5 left in my
> purse. It's more a case of 'God, I've got to pay back Monday what
> I borrowed from someone on Saturday.'   (p. 158)

Large-scale survey research also illustrates the hardship suffered by lone parents and their children. A survey of lone parents in 1993 found that almost half said that they worried about money 'almost all the time' (Ford *et al.* 1995).

As argued above, successive governments have had concerns about the increasing numbers of lone parents receiving income support, and corresponding increases in poverty. A consistent policy response has been to reform in-work benefits so that lone parents are better off in paid work than on Income Support. Family Income Supplement (FIS) was introduced in 1971 and was a means-tested benefit available to parents working 30 hours a week or more. In 1986, FIS became Family Credit and the number of hours was reduced in stages to 16 hours. In 1999, Family Credit was transformed into the Working Families Tax Credit. This was no longer a social security benefit but a tax credit. It would be paid through the wage packet rather than the benefit book. The government also made it available to people earning higher amounts of money than before. Further discussion of in-work benefits is in the final section of this chapter.

Overall, in-work benefits appear to have been successful in helping lone parents combine parenthood with paid work. In effect they allow lone parents to do a part-time job for a full-time wage. But there are some problems. For example, lone parents have no choice about payment method, they have to receive it through the wage packet and this may not be what they want. Also, when people move into work their eligibility for Housing Benefit will normally be reassessed and insecurity about this might discourage some people from getting a job in the first place. For those who do, the delays in reassessing a claim may cause financial difficulties.

The main categorical benefit for families is Child Benefit and this will be received by all lone parents, whether or not they are in paid work. This benefit is paid in recognition of the extra costs of having children, though the amount paid goes nowhere near meeting the full costs of having children. Some commentators argue that the best way to reduce poverty is to increase Child Benefit (and the child premiums on Income Support) and this appears to be close to the government's own current strategy (see the last section in this chapter).

The development of family benefits

Bieback (1992) has argued that benefits for families developed in three stages:

1.   Benefits for widows.
2.   Means-tested benefits including amounts for dependants.
3.   Benefits explicitly for children (such as Child Benefit).

These stages can be seen in the British system. Benefits for widows came first. Widows were often favourably treated under old systems of public assistance. They could receive 'outdoor relief' rather than having to enter the workhouse for support. The risk of widowhood was covered very early within insurance schemes. Widows' benefits were introduced as early as 1911 in Germany, 1926 in Britain. The state system enabled male workers to pay National Insurance contributions to provide insurance for their widows in the event of their death. The relatively favourable treatment of widows – compared with the separated or the divorced – continues in many social security systems today. They are covered from within the insurance, or contributory, elements of social security. The gendered nature of state provision is evident from the fact that, for the whole of the twentieth century, there was no provision for widowers; however, widowers with dependent children gained access to benefits from April 2001.

It has been argued that family benefits are a little separate from the traditional systems and functions of social security. Within a social assistance (means-test) approach, the prime aim is to alleviate poverty. This need not require any separate system for families. All those at risk of poverty will come within the scope of support. Within a social insurance approach, families have received little explicit recognition. Two issues are important here. First of all, there is the issue of who makes contributions to the National Insurance fund. Usually this is tied to paid work and so discriminates against women who spend more time working in the home than in the labour market. However, in the UK and Germany credits have been introduced to recognise caring responsibilities. So women who look after children can be credited with some insurance payments. The second issue to consider is the type of event or risk that insurance schemes are insuring people against. Generally these schemes insure people for retirement, unemployment and absence from paid work due to sickness/disability. The care of children – or of disabled or elderly relatives – has generally been excluded from the scope of such schemes. Instead this has often been viewed as a private matter – to be dealt with within families. Thus, again, women are unlikely to benefit from social insurance schemes (McLaughlin 1999).

Historically, family benefits have often been intended to help people cope with the extra costs of supporting children and therefore often focused on larger families (second or higher births). Pro-natalist factors (that is, the desire to increase the birth rate) may have been very important in some countries. For example, following the First World War, France was increasingly concerned that its population was declining at the same time as Germany's was increasing. The French were therefore keen to encourage women to have more children (Pedersen 1993).

Looking at the range of policies available to governments concerning lone parents, Kamerman and Kahn (1978) identified four key approaches:

1. Taking a mostly anti-poverty line (the UK), which will include a large degree of contact with lone parents.
2. Looking at single mothers as their own category (Norway).
3. Family policy is directed at young children in all families (France).
4. Integrating work and families (Sweden).

5.2 Lone parent families and poverty

We saw in Chapter 1 that lone parent families are overwhelmingly poor families. The social security system just outlined may reduce the depths of poverty that they would face in its absence but it currently provides little more than survival-level rations. This section reviews the extent and nature of lone parent poverty.

The extent of lone parent poverty

Of all children currently living in a lone parent family, nearly four in five have household incomes in the bottom 40 per cent of the income distribution (Department of Social Security 2000). So the majority live in low-income families. But what about poverty? There are many ways of measuring poverty but it is common to make a distinction between absolute poverty and relative poverty. This is a controversial area, with a strong literature of its own (see Alcock 1987, 1993, Spicker 1993 and Bradshaw 1999 for overviews). We do not intend to rehearse all these arguments here. However, at the present time, one of the most commonly cited benchmarks is to treat as 'poor' anyone living on an income that is below half the average (mean) income in the country. This is a measure of 'relative' poverty as it measures poverty relative to the income of all members of society.

The semi-official poverty line (now taken as below 60 per cent of median income) appears simple on the face of it but even this measure involves a great deal of complexity. For example, an important issue concerns how the needs of different sizes and types of family should be taken into account (Berthoud and Ford 1996). Clearly, a lone parent with two children needs more money than a single woman to live above any poverty threshold – but precisely how much more? And how are such differences in needs to be properly measured? In most empirical work, a system of 'equivalence scales' is used, that give different weighting to children of different ages, and to single people compared with couples. By and large, older children are assumed to require greater resources than younger children, to have the same standard of living. A single person is assumed to require about 60 per cent of the income of a couple to have the same living standard. So, incomes are often adjusted by measures giving different 'weight' to families of different size and with different composition.

Then there are questions about *whose* incomes should be counted. Should a lone parent family be treated as sharing in the living standard of the wider household in which it may be located (e.g. with grandparents or older, non-dependent, children) or can it be treated as a unit in its own right? Should there be any deductions made from income, such as to take account of housing costs? Another issue concerns whether or not poverty measures should be calculated 'before housing costs' or 'after housing costs'. This can make a considerable difference in levels of poverty and in making comparisons between different groups. Measures of poverty after housing costs come closer to including 'disposable' income in the calculation rather than merely total income. Those groups that generally receive more help with their housing costs, including lone parents, look better off after housing costs have been taken into account (compared with those who receive no help).

There are reports and statistics produced by the Department of Social Security that provide 'answers' to these questions, and other technical matters. It is worth bearing in mind that there are a large number of such questions that have to be dealt with. Issues of how to treat different families and sources of income are not just dry technical matters, but may considerably affect the adults and children who are regarded as being poor. And, therefore, the relative position of lone parents and their children within the overall income distribution.

According to the main published measure of low incomes (the Households Below Average Income – HBAI – figures), 62 per cent of children living in lone parent households live in poverty (in households with below half average income, after housing costs). This figure represents almost two children in three for lone parents and adds up to 1.8 million children living within lone parent families. The equivalent figure for all children is one in three (34 per cent) which adds up to about 3.8 million children. This means that taking all poor children together, about half (48 per cent) live in lone parent families. The main reason for the poverty-level incomes of lone parent families is related more to the lack of any earners, than to the fact of lone parenthood itself. Couples with children, where no one is working, fare about as badly as lone parent families in the income distribution.

Most poverty statistics (including the ones just quoted) assume that money is shared equally among members of the same household. In other words, each person in a given household is assumed to have the same standard of living. This will mean that everyone in the household is either above the poverty threshold or else everyone is below it. But research has shown that resources are not shared equally within the household and this means that not everyone in a household may share in its overall ('average') standard of living (Goode et al. 1998). Men in couples, particularly where they receive the main source of income themselves, may not share this income fairly with all other household members. If this is the case, then some women in households that appear to be 'average' could have spending power and possibly a living standard close to that of the 'poor'. Conversely, some men in 'poor' households could have spending power that was rather closer to the average.

Research in this area has highlighted differences in people's access to family income, and in the degree of control (or power) that is exercised over the distribution of income within the family. All of this can mean that women and children in couples face 'hidden poverty', perhaps to the extent that they might be better off in a lone parent family even though they would have lower household incomes. According to Land (1994), about a third of lone parents actually feel 'better off poorer' as lone parents. By this, it is meant that women who separate from a partner may actually be worse off in strict financial terms when they become a lone parent but they often feel better off because they have complete control over their income. Previously, some women would have only received partial, unpredictable and sometimes conditional access to the household's money and this can put them in an unbearable position. One of the women interviewed in a qualitative study by the authors (Rowlingson and McKay 1998) recalled that:

> Even though when you are in a couple I think you get more money, well we did get more money when we were in a couple, but it's him, he'd spend money like it was water. So I knew I would be better off without him.   (p. 160)

And another woman made a similar point:

> He used to get the giro and that was it, I wouldn't see any money.
>   (p. 161)

Questions about access to income, and power over its allocation, have so far been raised in relation to gender relations within the family. But the same questions should be raised about the distribution of income between adults and children, and between different generations of the same family sharing a household. It is generally assumed that parents, and mothers in particular, have the best interests of their children at heart and will go without things that they themselves need in order to provide items for their children. This is certainly what (lone) mothers tell us (Kempson *et al.* 1994) but the extent of this may vary considerably between families and we may get a different picture if we speak to children.

Even if a couple wish to share their resources fairly between themselves and their children, what would a fair distribution of resources be? This begs a more abstract question of how two different people (old and young, men and women) could be said to enjoy the same standard of living. Do men need more food than women, and if so, how much? Do children need more money spent on their leisure activities than their parents? And, if so, how much?

The methods used to measure poverty can provide descriptions of the numbers of families in poverty, the numbers of adults and the numbers of children. This should not disguise the fact that, as currently measured, children are considered to be poor because their parents are poor. As just discussed, there is no account taken of children who avoid poverty because their parents – usually their mothers – deprive themselves of essentials so that their children do not go without. Nor is much account taken of the possibility that children may not share in proportion to their needs in the resources of the families.

Policies to tackle poverty are therefore usually aimed at increasing the income of the household by getting more money to the parents. It is then assumed that this money will trickle down to the children. Another way of reducing child poverty might be to aim policies more directly at *children* by providing them with goods and services such as free school meals, free school uniforms, free school trips, free computers. As we shall see later in this chapter, the Sure Start programme comes within this category of tackling child poverty through a direct approach to children. But by and large policies currently aim to reduce child poverty through reducing the poverty experienced by families with children, and particularly through policies towards parents.

Lone parenthood and poverty: cause or effect?

What causes lone parent poverty? The most obvious answer is that the main cause of lone parent poverty is lack of employment (see Chapter 6), or employment on low earnings. This means that many lone parents have to rely on state benefits and these are set at low levels. This raises two further questions: why are benefits set at such a low level? And why do lone parents in Britain have low rates of participation in the labour market?

The first of these questions, relating to benefit rates, can best be explained by virtue of the dominance of capitalist free market interests. Those who accept the capitalist ideology of the free market believe that taxes and state spending should be as low as possible. In the UK this ideology is very strong compared with many continental European countries where ideologies of social inclusion are more important. Thus the UK has tended to keep taxation and spending much lower than continental European countries.

Turning to the second of these questions about the low employment rate of lone parents in the UK, a number of explanations can be put forward here. For example, lone parents in the UK have low levels of education and qualifications. Being mainly women from working-class backgrounds they can only find relatively low-paid work and may need to pay for childcare (and other in-work expenses) from relatively meagre earnings. Paid work may therefore not seem financially worthwhile compared with life on benefit. Lone parents may also buy into an ideology of motherhood that stresses the importance of mothers staying at home with their children. Even if paid work were financially worthwhile, they might still choose to stay at home with their children.

This is the classic argument and we might label this the 'lone parenthood as cause of poverty' argument. Many academics and policy-makers accept it. But the argument can be turned on its head. Perhaps lone parents are not only poor because of lack of employment but lack of employment and poverty leads them to become lone parents (see Chapter 1). We might call this the 'poverty as a cause of lone parenthood' argument. It is likely that lone parenthood is both a cause and effect of poverty rather than simply one or the other. For example, Hobcraft and Kiernan (1999) argue that childhood poverty begets early motherhood and adult poverty but that early motherhood also has a significant effect in increasing poverty.

It is also likely that the precise causal relationship between poverty and lone parenthood varies depending on the type of lone parent. For example, poverty is perhaps one of the main causes of single lone parenthood but it is less likely to be the cause of divorced lone parenthood (even though people from poor economic backgrounds are more likely to divorce; Ermisch 1991). Widowhood, too, is likely to have some link to prior poverty as ill health and death are unevenly distributed towards the bottom end of the income and class distribution.

5.3 Underclass, dependency and social exclusion

So far in this chapter we have argued that lone parent families are poor and that the social security system acts as a safety net, albeit a fairly ineffective one. The majority of lone parents receive means-tested benefits and this has led some commentators to say that they are part of an underclass. This section considers the arguments and the evidence in relation to debates about the underclass, dependency and social exclusion.

The underclass debate

The underclass debate has raged for a couple of decades now, fuelled repeatedly by the writings of Charles Murray (1996a, 1996b). There are many different definitions of the underclass but the underclass is usually said to consist of at least some of those people living on very low income for long periods. In many definitions (including Murray's), the attitudes and behaviour of the underclass are a necessary condition for membership of this group. These attitudes/behaviours include: little attachment to formal work (therefore unemployment or inactivity); lack of respect for the law (therefore crime and drug-taking); little attachment to marriage (therefore cohabitation and lone parenthood); and permissive sexual attitudes (therefore illegitimacy). Debate about the underclass is often heated and there is much disagreement about how it is defined, whether or not it exists, whether or not it is a useful concept, and what causes it to exist. While this is not the place to engage with all the debates, lone parents are at the centre of this debate and so some discussion is useful here.

Murray identifies three factors as associated with the underclass: crime; unemployment; and illegitimacy. He does not associate lone parenthood as a whole with the underclass, only single lone parenthood. It is unclear whether he includes cohabiting parents in his definition but he is certainly scathing of cohabitation and believes that marriage should be strongly supported by social and economic institutions. Murray argues that it is generally worse for children to be with one parent than with two and that children are more likely to be with one parent if they begin that way. The research evidence for this is unclear. The duration of lone parenthood is actually shorter for single lone mothers than it is for separated or divorced lone mothers (Rowlingson and McKay 1998). Murray appears to condemn the underclass but some passages could be used to argue for policies to tackle inequality and poverty so that people's education and life chances could be improved:

> When one leaves school without any job skills, barely literate, the job
> alternatives to crime or having a baby or the dole are not attractive.
> Young men who are subsisting on crime or the dole are not likely
> to be trustworthy providers, which makes having a baby without a
> husband a more practical alternative. (Murray 1996a: p. 48)

Murray's arguments and evidence have been criticised in a number of ways. His emphasis on single lone mothers is countered with the fact that these are a minority of all lone parents. But they are a growing group and the poorest of all lone parents. His argument that 'the children of single mothers do worse, often much worse, than the children of married couples' (1996a: p. 29) is echoed by others (Dennis and Erdos 1992) and is generally accepted but, once again, it is not completely substantiated by evidence (see Chapter 7).

Murray is prominent in the underclass debate, but other writers have employed the concept in different ways. Frank Field (1989) points to three groups as forming the underclass. These are: frail elderly pensioners; lone parents on benefit (thus including separated, divorced and even widowed lone parents as well as single lone mothers); and the long-term unemployed. He attributes four structural causes to the development of an underclass: unemployment; widening class differences; the exclusion of the very poorest from rising living standards; and a hardening of public attitudes. These factors have created a group of people who are separated from main-stream society in terms of income, life chances and political aspirations. Field places much less emphasis on attitudes and behaviour than Murray.

Other writers have formulated a more theory-driven conceptual-isation of the underclass. For example, Runciman (1990) uses class analysis to define the underclass as those beneath the working class who are per-manently excluded from the labour market. Smith (1992) takes a similar view defining the underclass as those with no stable relationship to the mode of production.

Murray's view is that the underclass have distinctive attitudes that contribute to their situation. This leads some writers to claim that Murray is 'blaming the victim'. But in a sense he does not blame the individuals – he argues that they are acting rationally according to the systems and structures they face. It is those systems and structures (including the social security system) that are the underlying cause of the attitudes and so should be changed. But do poor people have different attitudes to others in society? A range of studies (both qualitative and quantitative) have invest-igated the attitudes of poor people (including lone parents). These have found that poor people generally have the same attitudes and aspirations as the better off (Heath 1992, Kempson *et al.* 1994).

Dependency culture?

Difficulties in defining the underclass have led some to turn to the concept of 'dependency' on social security or social housing. Receipt of state benefits and/or social housing appears to be a much more straight-forward concept to operationalise than the underclass. However, the conditions under which receipt is then interpreted as dependence are still unclear. Most people (including some of the very richest) receive one or more state benefits (if we include the state retirement pension and Child Benefit). So the definition of dependence is generally narrowed to include only means-tested benefits. But some people receive means-tested benefits for a very short period of time so the definition tends to be narrowed to long-term benefit recipients. But how long is long-term? And what about the poorest groups (such as the homeless – or perhaps prisoners) who may not receive any benefits at all?

Whatever the precise definition, it is likely that lone parents would emerge as one of the main dependency groups. But the concept of dependency suggests that one group of people in society can be termed 'dependent' and another group 'independent'. In reality, all members of society are 'interdependent' to some extent. Some people are financially dependent on employers or the stock exchange or the property market or partners or parents. The term 'dependency' usually only refers to dependence on the state and this is seen as problematic in a way that other forms of dependency are not.

The term 'dependency culture' also suggests that people who are dependent on the state have different beliefs, values and behaviours compared with the rest of society. But as argued above, research does not provide any evidence of this.

Social exclusion

Notions of the 'underclass' and 'dependency culture' focus to a large extent on individual beliefs, values and behaviours. Commentators who take a more structuralist approach tend to employ the concept of social exclusion. It suggests that people are being excluded from mainstream society rather than voluntarily opting out. However, it still carries the connotation that those who are excluded are not part of mainstream society or culture and research suggests that this is the case only in so far as some people lack the opportunity to participate. They do not necessarily lack the desire to participate.

As with the concept 'poverty', there are many competing definitions of social exclusion (see Room 1995). At its heart, the term includes the following ideas:

- Relationships and participation – social exclusion involves people being excluded from participating in mainstream society.
- Multi-dimensionality – social exclusion is related to low skills, joblessness, poor health and poor housing.
- Dynamics and processes – social exclusion is usually seen as a process involving movements in and out of mainstream society.

In many ways, the term 'social exclusion' covers similar ground to the term 'deprivation' and in Chapter 9 we review the research on hardship

and deprivation faced by lone parent families. One reason for the adoption of the new term is that it is widely used in Europe (Room 1995).
European social policy has long taken an integrationist view of society –
focusing on issues of cohesion and social harmony. Indeed, European
policy-makers tend to talk more about social inclusion than social exclusion. British social policy and sociology has drawn slightly more from
a Marxist discourse stressing conflict and class cleavages. This has led to
a redistributive/egalitarian discourse but recently such a discourse has
given way to a social integration perspective. Levitas (1996: p. 5) argues
that the discourse in recent policy documents: 'treats social divisions
which are endemic to capitalism as resulting from an abnormal breakdown in the social cohesion which should be maintained by the division
of labour.'

In academic circles, the main definition of social exclusion involves
the idea that some people are excluded from participating in mainstream
society. This begs the question of what constitutes mainstream society.
And is it necessarily a bad thing if some people are outside it? The point
must surely be that people should have the power to choose whether
or not they wish to be part of the mainstream. This takes us back to a
discussion of people's resources (particularly their financial resources) as
it is from these that their power to choose a way of life will be largely
determined.

Recent government policy appears to equate 'participation in mainstream society' with 'participation in paid work'. They have advocated paid
work as the route out of poverty and social exclusion. Such an approach
places much less value on unpaid caring and community work. Levitas
(1996: p. 19) argues that 'what "integration" means is participation in a
capitalist economy driven by profit and based upon exploitation.' An alternative to the current government approach based on 'social exclusion as
exclusion from paid work' could be to increase benefits for those engaged
in socially useful tasks such as caring for children or other people.

There is no official measure of social exclusion but most measures
would probably include most lone parents as an excluded group.

5.4 Government strategy: tackling poverty and social exclusion

The Labour government elected in 1997 recognised, unlike the
previous government, that poverty existed and that it was a problem that
needed addressing by government. So how did this government address

the problem of poverty? It began quite early on with a commitment to eliminating child poverty within 20 years. In order to eliminate child poverty the government will inevitably have to tackle lone parent poverty. Children are considered to be poor if their parents are poor, and half of all poor children are in lone parent families. In 1998, the Department of Social Security produced a report that was sub-titled *A New Contract for Welfare*. This report outlined the government's general strategy and this can be summed up in their phrase: 'Work for those who can, security for those who cannot.'

Within the 'work for those who can' part of the strategy there are a number of agendas. The first of these (in the sense of being the most long-standing) is that of 'making work pay'. This is a continuation of the previous government's strategy that seeks to ensure that people who are in paid work see significant gains, in their income, from being in work, rather than not working and receiving benefit. The main flagship here is the new Working Families Tax Credit (WFTC) which replaced Family Credit in October 1999. Also within the 'Making Work Pay' agenda is the minimum wage and cuts to income tax for those in low-paid jobs. All these changes are likely to be particularly helpful to lone mothers, as it is these women who most often find themselves in low-paid work. The second agenda is 'welfare to work', which seeks to move people off benefit, and into paid work. The main schemes here are the various programmes each known as a New Deal (see Chapter 6 for further discussion of this scheme). Finally, there are various other agendas including those related to improving childcare and child support. These are intended both to make work pay and to make work possible.

As far as 'security for those who cannot' work is concerned, the government has recently increased the amount of money going to families with children that are not in paid work.

Box 5.1   Government strategy to reduce child poverty

- Making work pay – Working Families Tax Credit, minimum wage, income tax reform.
- Welfare to work – New Deal, ONE.
- National childcare strategy.
- Child support reforms.
- Child Benefit and Income Support reforms.

The 1970s–1990s: making work pay

During the 1970s and 1980s, governments took the view that it was for lone parents to judge whether or not paid work was best for them and their children. As such, lone parents have been able to receive Income Support, and other benefits, without the requirement to seek paid work. And there has been only limited emphasis on providing information or advice on what would happen to benefits on starting work. In fact, lone parents were able to continue receiving benefit with no work requirements until their youngest child was 16. This was highly unusual compared with most other countries where lone parents had work requirements far sooner. The USA is the classic example of a country where lone parents are required to work when their children are still babies (Waldfogel *et al.* 2001) but even countries as apparently pro-lone parenthood as Norway now stipulate that lone parents with children as young as three should be looking for, and taking, paid work (Skevik 2001). In the UK, the emphasis has been on policy measures within social security that have tried to make paid work more attractive and to remove potential barriers that lone parents might face in moving into paid work (and remaining there).

As mentioned earlier in this chapter, Family Income Supplement (FIS) was introduced in 1971 to provide a top-up for low-paid families with children working at least 30 hours a week. In 1988, FIS was replaced by Family Credit in an attempt to ensure that all families with children would be better off working than on Income Support. The scope of Family Credit was considerably extended in 1992, when the qualifying hours were reduced from 24 to 16 a week. This was particularly significant for lone parents, and indeed the most common number of hours worked by lone parents on Family Credit *is* 16. Other reforms were designed to help contribute towards the costs of formal childcare and to improve the attractions of paid work for those receiving maintenance (Inland Revenue WFTC statistics 2001).

In 1999, the year Family Credit ceased to exist, around 400,000 lone parents – or nearly one quarter of all lone parents, and over half those in paid work – received this benefit and other in-work benefits.

1999 onwards: making work pay – even more

In 1999, the Working Families Tax Credit (WFTC) replaced Family Credit. It incorporated several changes that increased the financial returns to paid work for lone parents (and couples with children). First of all, the rates of benefit were higher. There was a higher rate of support for adults, and higher rates of payment for children up to the age of 16. Therefore, in most cases families would receive more.

A second change was that, as a family's earnings rose, the effect on WFTC was less than for FC so the amount a family received in benefit would be reduced more slowly than before. Under FC, for each extra £1 that a family earned (take-home), FC awards were reduced by 70 pence. Under WFTC, each extra £1 in earnings reduces WFTC awards by only 55 pence.

Third, there was more help available within WFTC for childcare costs. This was partly because rates of support for childcare were higher, but also because childcare spending for some children of older ages was also admissible. As before, however, only 'formal' childcare arrangements (e.g. with registered childminders) would attract support. There continue to be debates about relaxing this limitation, to include financial support for family helpers, but no changes have been announced so far.

A final key reform has been in the treatment of maintenance (child support, alimony) payments. Previously, maintenance (apart from the first £15) was counted the same as extra earnings. This is to say that extra maintenance reduced the amount of FC received. However, *all* maintenance payments are disregarded in the calculation of WFTC. For lone parents receiving maintenance, work becomes more rewarding if their maintenance exceeds £15 each week. This may also provide more of an incentive for lone parents to pursue maintenance.

The negative side of WFTC, as some have seen it, is the general requirement for benefit to be paid through the wage packet. Family Credit was either paid by Order Book (slips of paper to be encashed at a local Post Office), or paid directly into bank or building society accounts. WFTC is paid into wage packets by employers, who are able to deduct such payments from their overall tax bill (or claim advance funds in certain circumstances). For lone parents, the likely problems of such a process are changes to their system of budgeting, and potential concerns about employers being aware of their overall financial and personal situation. On the basis of qualitative research with families, Goode *et al.* (1998) have suggested that payment to fathers might reduce the amount of money spent on children. Partly to meet such anxieties, applicants for WFTC are able to request that payment be made directly to non-working mothers.

Although changes to WFTC have been designed to increase the monetary advantages of paid work, some other benefit changes, however, may slightly reduce the financial incentive to do paid work. The rates of benefit for children under 11 are being raised, in a number of steps, to match the higher rates for children aged 11–15. Lone parents with children under 11 will gain by several pounds per week, per child, from this change.

Second, the proposed changes to child maintenance should mean that up to £10 of maintenance may be kept by those on Income Support. Previously, there was a pound for pound deduction for any maintenance received. However, the complete disregard of maintenance within WFTC should mean that there are still strong incentives for those receiving maintenance to take paid work.

A number of measures were announced in the 2001 budget to further increase the support for working families through WFTC. It was announced that this tax credit would be increased by £5 a week from June 2001. And there would be more help with childcare costs. Taken with increases in the minimum wage, the higher WFTC will mean that a family with one child who receives WFTC will be guaranteed to receive a minimum income of £214 a week from April 2001 rising to £225 a week in October. The amount of childcare costs that are eligible for this element of WFTC rises from £100 to £135 for one child, and from £150 to £200 for two children from June 2001 (*Financial Times*, 8 March 2001).

Easing the transition to work

Another more recent strand of reform was to improve the situation of lone parents (and others) at the *point of transition* from benefits into work. So the child maintenance bonus, and back to work bonus, could provide lump sums on returning to work. Housing Benefit and Council Tax Benefit could continue to be paid at previous levels, for a short time, on moving into work. More recently, Income Support may continue to be paid for two weeks for those lone parents taking paid jobs. From 2002, income support for mortgage interest will also be able to 'run on' when people return to work.

Welfare to work

As mentioned earlier, compared with most other Western countries, the UK has one of the most relaxed regimes as far as requiring lone parents to look for and take up paid work. This, however, is beginning to change, albeit rather slowly. The New Deal for Lone Parents (NDLP) provides personal advice and support to lone parents who have recently entered Income Support or are in the stock of existing Income Support claimants. The way NDLP works will be discussed in the next chapter. For the moment, we simply note that its main purpose is to help lone parents who wish to find a path back to employment, and that it is currently voluntary.

In 1999, the pilot 'ONE' programme (formerly known as the Single Work-Focused Gateway) began and this involved a still earlier intervention with lone parents (and other groups) who are initiating a benefit claim. In future, if legislation goes through, a policy of compulsory participation in the 'ONE' programme will be introduced. It is possible in the future that lone parents with children older than 5 years and 3 months will have to meet work requirements similar to those of other benefit claimants of working age.

National childcare strategy and child support reforms

The Labour government is committed to taking a 'joined-up' approach to policy, and in the field of child poverty it is approaching this through policies relating to childcare and child support.

During 1998 and 1999, the government progressively extended its National Childcare Strategy. This period saw a considerable increase in the provision of Out-of-School Clubs and a continuation of the trend to pre-school nursery classes for 3- and 4-year-olds. There is a commitment to train a further 50,000 childcare workers, through New Deal provision, and this should help to overcome a shortage of supply. Financial support for childcare in low-income working families is being addressed as part of the Working Families Tax Credit, discussed above.

The government is also trying to increase the amount of maintenance that lone parents receive from absent parents through reforms of the Child Support Act. These should in theory make lone parents better off whether in work or not (see Chapter 7 for further discussion).

Security for those who cannot work

So far most of these policies have been aimed at the first half of the overall strategy 'work for those who can'. What about security for those who cannot? The government got off to a poor start here. It had made a pre-election pledge to keep to the Conservative government's spending levels and so in 1997 it cut One Parent Benefit and the lone parent premium on Income Support. Those early cuts caused a great deal of controversy and were opposed by many within the Labour Party as well as within pressure groups for lone parents. The cuts are also likely to have damaged the morale of lone parents to the extent that they might not believe that the government has the best interests of lone parents at heart. But the 1999 and 2000 budgets raised levels of benefits for families with children (see p. 120).

A seamless system of financial support: Integrated Child Credit (ICC)

There are currently four sources of financial support for families with children: Child Benefit (an amount for each child paid to parents regardless of income or employment status); child allowances in Income Support (paid to non-working families); Working Families Tax Credit (paid to low/middle income families in employment); and the Children's Tax Credit (paid to all tax-paying families not paying higher-rate tax). In the 2000 budget, the government confirmed plans to reform this system. It plans to retain Child Benefit but to combine the other sources of support into a single payment to the parent caring for the child/ren – the Integrated Child Credit (see HM Treasury 2000). The aim of this reform is to provide a more stable and less complex system of support to families with children, particularly those on low incomes.

Research for the Joseph Rowntree Foundation (Hirsch 2000) argues that the success of these reforms will depend heavily on the detail of its design and delivery. This research has drawn lessons from similar systems in Australia, Canada and the USA and the main lessons are that systems are more successful if they are highly inclusive rather than focusing narrowly on those with lowest incomes. There is also a need to ensure that redistribution towards families with children is accepted as socially just. Finally the research argues that: the system must make sense to users; family payments must interact logically with other tax and benefit provision; and that they encourage rather than discourage people from doing paid work.

The 2001 budget was hailed a 'budget for families' by many commentators and the Chancellor of the Exchequer announced that the Children's Tax Credit would be received by all families where the chief wage-earner earns less than £50,000. This certainly makes the scheme fairly inclusive as it will be received by people high up the income scale.

Tackling social exclusion

Towards the end of 1997, the government set up a Social Exclusion Unit (SEU) to provide a joined-up approach to tackling social exclusion. The SEU has produced a number of reports about social exclusion but most of these have focused on fairly small 'problem groups' such as teenage mothers, truants, rough sleepers and 16–17-year-old 'NEETS' (those not in education, employment or training). It has not, therefore, considered the issue of social exclusion in a very broad sense. The government has also set up 18 policy action teams to consider particular aspects of social exclusion (such as financial exclusion and area regeneration) and further reports have been produced. Two of the main initiatives emanating from all this work (as far as lone parents are concerned) are the 'National strategy for neighbourhood renewal', which is closely linked to the New Deal for Communities, and the Sure Start programme.

The New Deal for Communities targets resources on some of the most deprived communities in Britain, many of which will have large populations of lone parents (Social Exclusion Unit 1998). But this was a fairly small scale exercise at first. In January 2001, the Prime Minister announced a pot of £131 million that communities could bid for over 3 years on top of £800 million already set aside as a neighbourhood renewal fund. The new money was intended to cover 88 local partnerships in the most deprived local communities (Social Exclusion Unit 2001). So although the scheme has been extended, it will still only cover a relatively small number of areas.

Another attempt to reduce social exclusion in deprived areas is the Sure Start scheme (Social Exclusion Unit 1998). This is a scheme, begun in 1998, for very young children in deprived areas (see Box 5.2) It is hoped that greater investment in the education of very young children in deprived areas should improve children's prospects. But the wider inequalities in society are not being addressed directly and so it is likely that we will continue to see poor women become poor lone mothers.

Box 5.2   Sure Start

- By 2002 there should be 250 Sure Start local programmes. These will be concentrated in areas where a high percentage of children are poor.

- It is funded to the tune of £452 million over three years.

- It is designed to improve local services for families with young children, such as through: home visiting; support for good quality play, learning and childcare experiences; advice about child health and development; personalised services for children and parents with special needs.

- Each local programme delivers a core set of services, but there is flexibility to provide extra services in line with local needs.

Source: Social Exclusion Unit (1998)

Evaluating the government's approach

Independent academics have estimated that all the policy changes announced by government from 1997 to January 2000 would take 840,000 children out of poverty (Piachaud and Sutherland 2000). This amounts to about a quarter of all children in poverty at the start of this period. The changes would also reduce the depth of poverty (the poverty gap) by about a quarter. In 1999 and 2000, the government's budgets were particularly generous to families with children. For example, Child Benefit was increased substantially and in the 2000 budget it also announced increases to income support of £4.35 per week per child under 16. With all these measures the government expects to take a total of 1.2 million children out of poverty by the end of 2001 (Gordon Brown's March 2000 budget speech).

Government changes will take substantial numbers of children out of poverty. And its commitment to tackling poverty and social exclusion should improve the lives of lone parent families quite substantially. Those out of work have seen their incomes rise (though they are still relatively poor). Those in work have also seen their incomes rise. This all sounds good, and represents a significant first step towards reducing child poverty. But it still means that the majority of today's poor children will still be poor – there will still be 2 to 3 million children left in poverty even if these policies are successful (for example, if there is no recession). And it is likely that those children taken out of poverty will be those most easily rescued from deprivation. The more difficult cases will be left. So let's take a more critical look at the government's strategy.

In line with most government policy that tries to move people (back) into paid work, the government's approach to lone parents is to concentrate on providing encouragement and financial incentives to individuals. It is therefore a 'supply-side' approach, focusing on the supply of labour. It does little to stimulate demand for labour in inner cities and other parts of the country where demand is still relatively low (see Chapter 9).

Another reason why current government policy is unlikely to be successful in this field is that, to some extent, it flies in the face of what lone parents themselves want to do. Many lone parents see themselves as mothers first and workers second (as do many mothers in couples). For government to be successful in encouraging lone parents into paid work it will have to be accompanied by a culture shift in which mothers increasingly identify themselves as workers rather than mothers.

Another limitation of the government's policy is that the whole strategy is based on the 'lone parenthood as cause of poverty' argument.

It does not address the more fundamental issues that are posed by the 'poverty as cause of lone parenthood' argument. Having said that, if current lone parents become better off, this could have a second-order effect of providing their children with better experiences and opportunities. Poverty and inequality are fundamental issues that need to be tackled more directly, for example, with greater redistribution of resources through the tax and benefit systems.

5.5 Summary

We have already established the clear links between poverty and lone parenthood. By all conventional definitions and measures, most lone parent families are poor. According to official figures, about two-thirds of children living in lone parent families are poor. This adds up to about 1.8 million children. We have highlighted, however, that these conventional definitions and measures have various limitations, especially when applied to lone parent families. None of these limitations question the basic conclusion that lone parent families are generally poor families but they do cause us to stop and think about how we measure poverty and living standards within these families.

The association between poverty and lone parenthood is clear but does this association occur because lone parenthood causes poverty or because poverty causes lone parenthood? We argue that both mechanisms are at work but affect different types of lone parents to different extents.

One of the main methods by which the state attempts to alleviate (rather than prevent) lone parent poverty is through the social security system. One of the problems for lone parents is that over half of them are having money deducted from their basic income support payments, mostly in order to replay loans from the social fund. So lone parents are living on even less than basic safety net levels of income.

The increasing numbers of lone parents on benefit have led successive governments to consider ways of reducing this expenditure. In-work benefits have been made more and more generous in order to tempt lone parents (back) into paid work. Family Income Supplement was introduced in 1971 followed by Family Credit in 1986 and Working Families Tax Credit in 1999. Prior to the introduction of WFTC in 1999, 20 per cent of lone parent families were receiving Family Credit. This benefit was means tested and was available to low-income lone parents working at least 16 hours a week.

The level of poverty among lone parent families, together with their rate of receipt of means-tested benefits has led some commentators to talk of their part in an underclass. Murray has been most active in discussing the nature of the underclass and he includes single mothers within this group.

Another set of debates revolves around the concept of 'social exclusion' and this term has become widely used in government and academic circles. In many ways, it is similar to the concept of 'deprivation' though it has built on more recent research that has analysed the dynamics of poverty and inequality. Social exclusion occurs when some people are excluded from mainstream society, though recent government applications of this term appear to equate exclusion from mainstream society with exclusion from paid work.

Paid work is no guarantee of a route out of poverty, but this is the route that recent governments have encouraged people to follow. In the 1970s and 1980s, governments were keen to 'make work pay' by introducing and reforming in-work benefits. In 1997, following a massive rise in child poverty, the new government promised to eradicate child poverty. Welfare-to-work became the clarion call. A multitude of 'New Deals' were spawned including one specifically for lone parents. The new government was determined to make work pay – even more than the previous governments. Working Families Tax Credit was introduced in 1999. There were also reforms of childcare provision and child support. For those still on benefit, the government eventually decided to increase levels of benefit.

The only immediate way to reduce poverty is to raise benefit levels substantially, a step that the government is reluctant to take. Its reluctance can be explained partly because of its fear of being seen as a 'tax and spend' party. But it is also the case that the government has an ideological commitment to paid work as the best way out of poverty and there would be less financial incentive to work if benefit levels were higher.

chapter 6

Work and employment

As we saw in Chapter 1, lone parents in Britain are much less likely to have paid jobs than those in most other countries. They are also much less likely to work than all mothers in couples, with the difference particularly marked for part-time work. This low rate of employment is partly because lone parents have relatively little education and few qualifications, and reflects the fact that lone parents often have young children. But whatever the reasons for this low rate, the government is currently trying to increase the proportions of lone parents in paid employment. It sees employment as the best way of improving the living standards of lone parents and their children. In the past, however, it was often considered best for children if their mother stayed at home and cared for them. And indeed, when benefits for lone parents were introduced in the 1930s in the USA, they required lone parents to stay at home. The equivalent benefits today are more likely to be used to compel them to take paid work. Thus there is a tension between the roles of 'mother' (as child-carer) and 'worker'. The nuclear family of past years was thought of as containing both a worker and a carer: with lone parents there is often a conflict between which of these two roles is seen as the priority.

This chapter begins with a discussion of gendered perspectives on work to show how paid work in the labour market (the public sphere) is increasingly valued by the state above unpaid work in the home (the private sphere). It then looks at the type of work carried out by lone parents in employment before revisiting the question of why relatively few lone parents in Britain currently have paid jobs. The chapter then reviews the New Deal and other policies designed to encourage lone parents to move into paid work. It ends with a discussion of the pros and cons of working (lone) motherhood.

6.1 Work, gender and the free market

Views and policies about lone parents and work are heavily affected by 'common sense' notions of work. These notions are both highly gendered and also highly coloured by free market philosophy. The following example illustrates both these points. Two women could be living next door to each other. One is a lone mother who is looking after three children of her own. Her only source of income is from social security benefits. Her next-door neighbour is also a lone mother who is looking after one child of her own and two children of a friend of hers. She receives money from her friend and a top-up social security benefit called Working Families Tax Credit (see Chapter 5). Both women are looking after the same number of children and are doing virtually the same things each day but one is generally seen to be 'working' while the other is not. And the second mother will have a much higher income than the first. This is solely because the second is receiving some of her income from a non-state source and is not totally reliant on benefits. Our views about 'work' therefore tend to hide the amount of labour that women do in the home and with their children. As Grint (1991: p. 12) argues: 'the difference between work and non-work seldom lies with the actual activity itself . . . what counts as work cannot be severed from the context within which it exists.' The 'context' in most cases is the free market.

The work that women do in the home and with their children is often unpaid. It lies outside the formal labour market. The state, to date, has given some limited recognition to the work that women do in the form of benefits such as child benefit and income support (see Chapter 5). Child Benefit is paid direct to all mothers in recognition of the extra costs associated with children. Income Support is paid to lone mothers not working 16 hours a week or more, but similar benefits are also available to couples who are part of non-working families with children. Until the late 1990s there was little discussion about compelling lone parents receiving income support to look for, or be available for, paid work. Their role in looking after their children was considered sufficiently valuable in itself. However, the 'value' placed on this has been relatively low as income support is set at very low levels. But the government was wary of compelling mothers to take paid jobs.

Notions about women and work vary over time and between countries. During the Second World War, women were drawn into the factories and the Land Army. The government massively increased the numbers of nurseries and crèches to facilitate this friendly invasion of women into paid work. After the war, the nurseries were closed down. Women were expected (and in some cases compelled) to leave their jobs on marriage. Kiernan *et al.* (1998: p. 242) report that within a year of the war the number of day nurseries in England and Wales were reduced from 1,300 to 914 and by the mid-1950s there were little more than 20,000 places compared with over 70,000 places at their peak.

Mothers in the immediate post-war period were expected to care for their children at home. Evidence suggests that most women were happy to return to the home and make way for their husbands to take over the paid jobs. Pro-natalist sentiments emphasised the important role of women in having and bringing up children. Motherhood was assigned some status (but little power). Research by Bowlby (1951) strongly reinforced the idea that mothers should be with their pre-school children full-time. If they were not, research suggested that children would suffer severe emotional disturbance. This research has now been put back into the narrow context from which it originally emerged (see later in this chapter for a review) but, at the time, it was highly influential and it still resonates today. And even once children went to school, the spectre of 'latchkey children' was used to discourage women from placing paid work too high in their priorities. Work might be tolerated so long as children were unaffected by it. Mothers in poor families who 'needed' to work for money were criticised as were mothers from better-off families who 'chose' to work for money and/or self-fulfilment. Children were meant to come first and in the decades immediately after the Second World War, it was thought that this entailed women staying in the home with them. At the very most, women might consider part-time work if this fitted in around school timetables.

But the demands of capitalism began to undermine these patriarchal assumptions. In the 1950s there were labour shortages, particularly in the public sector such as in education, health and welfare. Ethnic minorities were encouraged to migrate to Britain to fill these jobs and women were also considered an important 'reserve army' of labour. From 1900 to 1930, the proportion of women in paid work was about one in ten. In 1955, it was about 22 per cent and by 1981 it had increased to about half (Grint 1991: p. 215). So by the early 1980s more and more married women, and mothers, remained in, or returned to, work but there were still strong cultural norms dictating that mothers should only work around their children's schooling, and not generally while children were of pre-school age.

British culture remains highly ambivalent about working mothers. Mothers are often expected to work if their family needs extra resources (to supplement a husband's in the case of married women, or to provide the sole income, in the case of lone parents). But the impact on children is still a cause of concern for some. And there is ambivalence towards 'career women' who provide the main (or equal) resources in a couple or, in the case of lone parents, see paid work as similarly important to work in the home. To a large extent, women appear to have accepted these general ideologies of motherhood. Research suggests that they like the opportunity to do part-time work (even if it is low-paid) because it fits in with the work they also wish to do in the home. Duncan and Edwards (1997) talk of the 'gendered moral rationalities' of lone parents that dictate their decisions about paid work. Thus lone mothers are not making decisions based on narrow economic rationality but on the basis of social norms relating to cultural expectations of motherhood.

This has led Hakim (1991) to coin the highly controversial term 'grateful slaves' for women, including lone parents, who work in low-paid, low-status, part-time work. Other researchers (see Walby 1986, Crompton and Sanderson 1990) stress the structural inequalities and discrimination that have created such work, and positioned it as 'women's work'. Capitalist and patriarchal structures and assumptions confine most women to the secondary labour market which contains much poorer jobs than the primary labour market. Thus women, lone mothers among them, have little choice but to engage with poor jobs if they wish to engage with the labour market at all.

While attitudes and behaviour in relation to women's work have changed to some extent, attitudes and behaviour in relation to 'men's work' have altered very little. Men are still expected to be the main breadwinners, even though fewer are able to fulfil that role these days. And research has shown that, even where women have moved into paid work, men in couples are not picking up a higher share of work in the home (Kiernan 1992). Childcare and housework are still seen as the 'natural' work of women. Some 'new men' may have begun to do a little more of the childcare and housework but there is still a long way to go. This leaves working women with the 'double burden' of having to do paid work outside the home and unpaid work in the home. Reeves (2000) argues for equal employment rights for men in the field of parenting. He argues that men will only start to identify themselves as carers if the law around maternity/ paternity rights gives equal benefits to men as it does to women. It is true that the law currently reinforces the view that women should be the main carers. Changes in the law might change men's views and behaviour to some extent but this will come at a cost for the state. Should this extra money be spent on men who *might* pick up more of the caring work or on women whom we know are currently doing that work? If we knew for sure that men would take on more of the work, then such a change in the law might be considered a positive one, but if they do not do so, then the change in law will be a failure at the expense of women and the state in general.

Another way of tackling the issues around men's roles in relation to childcare might be to encourage more men to apply for jobs as carers or teachers in nurseries and primary schools. At the moment these jobs are primarily filled by women and this serves to reinforce the identification of women with caring to the exclusion of men. But men are unlikely to apply for such jobs while rates of pay and levels of status are so low (see Land 2001).

6.2 Lone parents in paid work

The first section of this chapter has considered the relationship between gender, work and the free market. What is the outcome of this for lone parents? In 1999, about two lone parents in five were working 16 hours a week or more (Marsh *et al.* 2001). Lone fathers, widows and ex-married mothers were more likely to be in paid work and this was at least partly related to the age of the youngest child. These groups were less likely than others to have very young children, and those with very young children were less likely to work.

As we saw in Chapter 1, compared with other countries, Britain has a low level of employment participation among lone parents. And this level has declined in recent years. As Figure 6.1 shows, from 1979 to 1981, 49 per cent of lone mothers were in paid work (Bryson *et al.* 1997). By 1990–92, this figure had declined to 41 per cent. The trend for all mothers was in the opposite direction (from 52 per cent in 1979–81 to 62 per cent in 1990–92). This means that there is now a much higher rate of participation in paid work among all mothers compared with lone mothers. This divide is new, significant and, in comparative context, unusual. In 1979–81, almost a quarter (23 per cent) of lone mothers worked full-time compared with 17 per cent of all mothers. By 1990–92, that picture had totally reversed so that full-time work was more common among all mothers than it was among lone mothers.

Employment is often hailed (by the current government in particular) as a means of escaping poverty and social exclusion and so the decline in lone parents' participation rates is often a source of concern. However, Britain has a fairly low wage economy and lone parents often find themselves in low-paid work. This reflects the general position of women in the workplace where there is both vertical (occupational) and horizontal (job

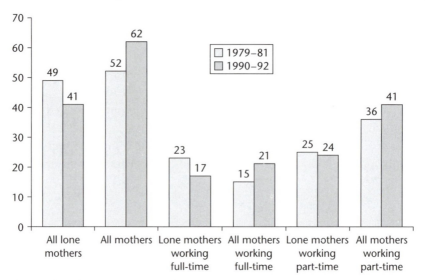

Figure 6.1 Employment participation among mothers.

Source: Bryson *et al.* (1997)

grade) gender segregation. This means that women are generally concentrated in particular occupations, including catering, cleaning, retail and services. These types of jobs are generally low paid compared with 'men's' occupations. Women are also concentrated in the jobs at the bottom of the job hierarchy in any particular field they work in. So both vertical and horizontal segregation combine to place women in the worst jobs. Lone parents, being mostly women from poor backgrounds, are even more confined to the poorest jobs, as we shall see.

In 1999, the majority (61 per cent) of lone parents who were working 16 hours a week or more were in jobs that qualified them for state assistance (Family Credit as it was then). Family Credit was set at a sliding scale and so it is available to people on moderate incomes as well as those on very low incomes but it is an indicator of the level of pay received by lone parents. Almost half (47 per cent) of lone parents working 16 hours a week or more were receiving Family Credit, the remaining 14 per cent were eligible but not receiving the benefit. Around one in three (32 per cent) were above the levels of earnings which qualify people for Family Credit (Marsh *et al.* 2001).

So far we have just looked at those working over 16 hours a week but it is interesting to make a distinction between working 16–29 hours a week ('part-time') and 30 hours a week or more ('full-time'). Working lone parents in 1999 were almost equally divided between those working part-time (48 per cent) and those working full-time (52 per cent). Hours of work were strongly correlated with income. Those working full-time were far more likely to be on moderate or high incomes – above the levels at which they could have been entitled to Family Credit (Marsh *et al.* 2001), with high incomes defined as being at least 35 per cent above this level.

Income was also associated with the type of work lone parents were engaged in. In 1999, most lone parents worked in the service sector – 43 per cent worked in unspecified services including health, education and public administration. A further 26 per cent worked in retail, hotel and catering. High income was positively associated with unspecified services but negatively associated with retail, hotel and catering. Only just over a quarter of all lone parents were in managerial or professional/associate professional jobs, compared with over half of all lone parents on high incomes.

Marsh *et al.* (2001) have constructed a 'quality index' for jobs based on the following indicators:

- Hourly net wage rates.
- Whether or not there is managerial/supervisory duty.
- Whether the job is permanent or temporary.
- Trade union membership.
- Membership of an occupational pension scheme.
- Training received, its type and duration.

As we can see from Table 6.1, short hours and low incomes went together with poor-quality jobs.

Table 6.1 Job quality by type of worker

Indicator	All working 16 hours or more	Family Credit recipient (low income)	High income	Part-time (16–29 hours)	Full-time (30 hours or more)
Median hourly wage rate (£)	4.40	3.88	7.48	4.00	5.02
Manager	14	4	40	4	23
Permanent job	92	91	95	90	94
Member of trade union	26	14	52	19	34
Member of occupational pension scheme	39	20	73	22	54
Received training	43	31	67	34	34

Source: SOLIF 1999 (Marsh *et al.* 2001: Table 9.7)

Table 6.1 shows that Family Credit recipients and part-time workers have a similar jobs profile (as we might expect because these two categories overlap to a large extent). They have lower hourly wages than average and are highly unlikely to have managerial responsibility. They are less likely to be members of trade unions or occupational pension schemes. And they are less likely than average to have received training. Those in high-income jobs do far better on all these indicators. Those in full-time jobs also do better on these indicators but not to the same extent as the high earners.

6.3 Lone parents not in paid work

As we have seen, the majority (62 per cent) of lone parents were not working 16 hours a week or more in 1999. However, we must remember to qualify this by saying that these parents were looking after their home and family, a job in itself, though unpaid. The government is keen to increase the numbers in paid work so why are so many lone parents currently out of paid work? And how keen are they to find a paid job?

As shown in Table 6.2, in 1999, one lone parent in five was out of work but had some current attachment to the labour market (either looking for a job or working less than 16 hours or expecting to look for a job soon). These lone parents will form the immediate target group for government policy. A further one in three had a much looser attachment

Table 6.2 Lone parents' attachment to the labour market in 1999

	All lone parents
In the labour market:	
Working 16+ hours a week	38
Strongly attached to the labour market:	
Currently looking for work	10
Working less than 16 hours	5
Expecting to look soon	6
Loosely attached to the labour market:	
Expect to look some time in the future	32
No/little attachment:	
Don't know when will look	4
Don't expect to look	5

Source: SOLIF 1999 (Marsh *et al.* 2001: Table 8.3)

Table 6.3 Reasons for not working among non-working lone parents in 1999

	All lone parents in 1999
Already looking for full-time job	7
Don't want to spend more time away from children	27
Affordability of childcare	23
Availability of childcare	16
Own illness/disability	16
Better off not working	10
Child's illness/disability	7
Don't have the skills	6
Studying/on a training scheme	6
Retired	5
Would be unable to pay rent/mortgage	3
Other family illness	2
No work available	2
Pregnant	1

Source: SOLIF 1999 (Marsh *et al.* 2001: Table 8.6)

to work, saying that they expected to look for a job some time in the future but have no immediate plans. The task of policy here would be to try to bring that date forward. A further one in ten had little or no attachment to work (Marsh *et al.* 2001). Other studies (Bradshaw and Millar 1991, Hales *et al.* 2000b) show similar levels of attachment to work.

A postal survey of around 600 lone mothers receiving Income Support found high rates of attachment to paid work, for both financial and other reasons (Noble *et al.* 1998). Attitudes to work were also more positive among younger mothers on Income Support.

Why are so few lone parents in paid work (compared with mothers in couples and lone parents in other countries)? Table 6.3 shows the reasons lone parents give for not looking for a paid job of 16 hours a week or more. Some lone parents (7 per cent) are looking for such but most are not and the main reason given for not doing so is that they do not want to spend more time away from their children (27 per cent). The afford-ability and availability of childcare are also frequently cited answers (by 23 per cent and 16 per cent respectively). Illness/disability is the next most important barrier to work (quoted by 16 per cent in relation to their own illness/disability, 7 per cent in relation to their child's and 2 per cent in relation to some other person's). A finding that is rather worrying for government policy is that 10 per cent said that they think they are better off not working and a further 3 per cent said that they would not be able to pay the rent or mortgage if they worked full-time. This shows either that the government's attempts to 'make work pay' are failing or they are simply not recognised by lone parents.

The following sections of this chapter review some of the explanations given by lone parents for not working full-time. They also consider why employment rates of lone parents went down over the 1980s and early 1990s.

Orientations to work and social expectations

The most common reason given by lone parents for not looking for work in 1999 was that they did not want to spend more time away from their children (Marsh *et al.* 2001). These people primarily identified themselves as parents (usually mothers) rather than workers. In the past, such a view chimed with the sentiments of society in general and government in particular. Now, however, government is keen to re-orientate lone parents towards work.

There is sometimes concern (usually expressed as part of the dependency debate) that lone parents are happy to be receiving state benefits and do not place great value on paid work. But there was no evidence from the survey by Marsh *et al.* (2001) to support such a view. About three-quarters of all lone parents agreed that 'having a job is the best way for me to be an independent person'. And even if we focus on the group most often referred to in the dependency debate – the non-employed, single never-married lone mothers – a majority (58 per cent) also agreed with the statement. On a range of attitudinal statements there was very little difference between lone parents in work and lone parents not in work. This supports the view that non-working lone parents are out of work because of their situations (such as having young children). They feel that they should care for their children personally rather than take on paid work. They are positive about employment but only when it does not interfere with their roles as mothers.

The views of lone parents in 1999 were generally very similar to those of mothers in low-income couples (Marsh *et al.* 2001). Surprisingly perhaps, lone parents were slightly less likely than mothers in couples to agree that 'a job is alright but I really want to be with my children at home.' This further reinforces the point that there was no evidence to suggest that the reason why lone parents are less likely to work than mothers in couples is due to differences in attitudes.

Can orientations to work explain the declining rate of employment of lone parents? Orientations are certainly important but, on their own, they cannot explain the declining employment rate. If anything, women's views about work are becoming more positive rather than less so it is difficult to believe that lone parents recently became more home-orientated.

Childcare

Childcare has long been seen as an important barrier to work according to lone parents. It is difficult for some lone parents to find childcare and it is particularly difficult to find affordable childcare. The average hourly price of paid childcare is higher in Britain than in any other European Union country, and in the mid-1990s it was estimated that a lone parent with low earnings capacity and no unpaid childcare help could be £60 per week worse off in work than out of work, even after in-work benefit payments (Bradshaw *et al.* 1996). This is quite different from the situation of most male unemployed job-seekers, who would generally be much better off in work than on Jobseeker's Allowance. As we shall see, the state now gives lone parents much greater support towards the costs of childcare but it is likely that childcare is still a barrier to employment for many lone parents (Ford 1996).

Accordingly, lone parents in employment in Britain have tended to consist largely of two groups: those with high earnings capacity, who can afford paid childcare, and those with unpaid childcare support or with all their children at secondary school. Unpaid childcare support has tended to be limited because of a background of family disruption: for example, only one in five lone mothers has the support of her own parents or in-laws (Marsh *et al.* 2001).

While childcare is certainly an important issue in relation to the absolute levels of paid work among lone parents, it is difficult to see how childcare issues can wholly explain decreasing employment rates of lone parents. Formal childcare seems to be becoming more widespread as demand for it generally increases. The supply of informal childcare may be declining slightly, however, as 'grandmothers' are more likely than those in former generations to be working themselves.

Illness or disability

For those with little or no attachment to work, a key factor was illness or disability. In the 1999 survey, half of those who did not expect to look for work in the future said that this was because they were ill or disabled. There is some evidence that levels of illness or disability among lone parents have increased (see Chapter 9) but not to the extent that would explain reduced labour market participation.

Education and qualifications

Relatively few lone parents said that lack of skills was a reason why they were not working more than 16 hours a week but lone parents have low levels of education and training and this severely affects their chances of finding work, particularly work that is well-paid. As shown in Chapter 1, almost three-quarters of lone parents had left school at 16 or under. Only 8 per cent remained in education beyond 18. Those (albeit relatively few) lone parents with high incomes (meaning at least 35 per cent above Family Credit levels) were half as likely as average to have left school before 16 (35 per cent compared with 73 per cent). And they were almost eight times more likely than average to have remained in education beyond 18 (35 per cent compared with 8 per cent). So high income seems strongly correlated with education.

Qualifications, too, are strongly correlated with income. A third of lone parents (37 per cent) had no academic qualifications and this percentage was highest for those out of work (44 per cent). But only 7 per cent of the high-income group had no qualifications. Only 6 per cent of all lone parents had degrees but 38 per cent of high-income lone parents had such qualifications.

Vocational qualifications were more common among lone parents. Almost half (45 per cent) had one or more vocational qualifications. These qualifications were most common among those on moderate incomes.

One way of improving levels of job participation is therefore to increase the level of education and qualifications of lone parents. And new initiatives are beginning to improve the educational prospects of disadvantaged young women – such as through the New Deal for Young People, as well as that for lone parents. Such initiatives may have additional effects in reducing the number of young women who become lone parents if, as argued in Chapter 3, low levels of education are a factor contributing to the reason why some young women become lone mothers.

Financial disincentives

Research has shown that financial factors are important in lone parents' choices to become employed or to remain on Income Support (Bryson *et al.* 1997). These choices are dominated on the one hand by the levels of out-of-work income available to the lone parent, and on the other hand by the earnings capacity of the lone parent if in employment and the childcare costs that would arise in that case. In the past, the benefit system has weakened financial incentives to work: some lone parents could have seen their income drop if they moved into paid work. However, during the 1980s, the average level of benefit payments fell substantially in relation to average earnings or average income. This change, combined with the increasing generosity of in-work benefits such as Family Credit should have led to increasing participation in work among lone parents but, on the contrary, there was a decline.

Perhaps lone parents are unaware of all the help provided to them in work or perhaps they know from experience that, despite the reforms, the reality means that they are still not better off in work. Another possibility is that, even if they are better off in work in a strict financial sense, the extra stress and the double burden of unpaid work in the home on top of paid work outside make any extra money seem barely worth it. And even if they were much better off in paid work, perhaps lone parents' identities as 'mothers first' prevent them from considering becoming workers. Perhaps government could provide free childcare places and enormous financial incentives but these might still fail to shake the priorities of some lone parents.

General rise in unemployment and wage inequality

The 1980s saw a general rise in unemployment that might explain increasing numbers of lone parents out of work but this hypothesis cannot explain why their employment declined in relation to other women and other mothers who face similar economic conditions.

Another trend during the 1980s, however, might provide a partial explanation. At this time, there was a widening wage gap between the low-paid and those on average pay levels. Lone parents tend to be in the lowest-paid jobs and so may have had less and less incentive to take the increasingly poorly paid work at their end of the jobs market.

Changes in the composition of lone mothers

The most convincing argument used to explain declining employment rates among lone parents relates to the changing composition of lone mothers. The proportion of lone mothers with very young children has been rising considerably, reflecting the growth in the number of single lone mothers, and these types of lone parents have always had much lower employment participation rates than others (Dilnot and Duncan 1992).

The link between age of youngest child and employment participation occurs for a number of reasons. For example, the age of the youngest child will affect some of the factors mentioned above. Society expects parents of pre-school children to be carers primarily and this will affect orientations to work among this group. Also, childcare for babies and toddlers is more scarce and more expensive than childcare for 3–4-year-olds or older children. More fundamentally, the types of lone parent who have very young children are often those from particularly poor backgrounds. These women have even lower levels of education and qualifications than lone parents on average and so find it most difficult to get worthwhile jobs. There is therefore a vicious circle whereby poor educational and employment opportunities contribute to the creation of lone parent families which then compound poor educational and employment opportunities.

The declining rate of employment among lone parents is therefore driven by the changing composition of the group. The changing composition then has implications for orientations to work, childcare, educational qualifications and skills of lone parents, and poor employment prospects.

6.4 Policies to encourage lone mothers to take paid work

As we have just seen, lone parents face a number of barriers to work. Two of the main barriers (which are related) are the financial disincentive to work which many face and the difficulties finding suitable and affordable childcare. The National Childcare Strategy aims to remove some of the barriers relating to childcare while the Working Families Tax Credit increases financial assistance with childcare for lower-paid lone parents through the Childcare Tax Credit. The more pervasive barrier is the nature of lone parents' orientations to work. Many simply do not feel ready to look for paid work and those that do may have last worked some time ago. This issue is being tackled by the New Deal for Lone Parents which is the most significant recent policy change in relation to lone parents. This initiative must be set in the broader policy context of 'Work for those who can, security for those who cannot' (see Chapter 5). However, it is not entirely clear how this slogan applies to lone parents – can they work or not? This is a complex and emotive issue. Of course most lone parents (but not all) are physically/mentally able to work but should we expect them or force them to get a paid job, and in what circumstances? The main issue here is usually the age of the children. It is more acceptable to expect lone parents with school-age (particularly secondary school-age) children to work than those with pre-school-age children. But the health of the children may also be considered an important factor. This issue is debated later in this chapter.

Before focusing on the New Deal scheme in Britain (and putting it into the context of other similar schemes around the world) it is important to mention another area of policy regarding employment. This is the extent to which parents (whether lone parents or couple parents) are provided with support to maintain themselves in employment. For example, much has been said recently about making it easier for parents to combine work and family life through increasingly flexible employment practices. But how far are these a reality? And how far does the state help out here?

Support for the work-life balance

Much has recently been said about helping parents to combine employment and family life. The Department of Trade and Industry (2000) recently launched a consultation paper on the subject with the Secretary of State making it clear that the needs of parents and children must be considered alongside the needs of employers. Land (2001) points out that one of the most important issues for parents in terms of combining employment and family life is the length of the working day. In some countries, there are policies designed to reduce the working week (e.g. to 35 hours for all in France and 32 hours a week for parents in the Netherlands). The aim in the Netherlands is to encourage the 'combination scenario' of both parents (in couples) sharing both paid work outside the home with unpaid work within the home. There is no explicit policy on hours of work for lone parents. The UK had the highest average weekly hours of work for full-time employees in the EU in the late 1990s (Office of National Statistics 2000). The EU Working Time Directive has improved the situation slightly in the UK, particularly in terms of the rights of part-time employees and shift-workers.

As well as looking at terms and conditions of employment, the work–family life balance is also aided through rights to parental leave. Maternity and parental leave are now rights in EU countries but there are considerable variations between member states in terms of the length of leave and the level at which it is paid, if at all. Scandinavian countries are far more generous in terms of both the length of leave and the level. Some countries, including Norway, specify that the father must take some of the leave or it is lost. The USA and Australia have much worse parental leave arrangements – with no paid parental leave. The UK stands in the middle of these two with some paid leave but nowhere near as generous as the Scandinavian countries (Land 2001).

The March 2001 budget announced a number of measures to improve family life in general, including around maternity and paternity leave. The current £60.20 flat-rate maternity pay will rise to £100 a week by 2003 when the period of leave covered will be extended from 26 weeks from the present 18. In addition, all new fathers will get the right to two weeks' paid paternity leave. And there is an increase in the sure start maternity grant (paid to low-income parents) from £300 currently to £500 next year.

Another aspect to the work–family life balance is the right to return to part-time work after the birth of a child. In the UK, USA and Australia, neither mothers nor fathers have an absolute right to return to work part-time following the birth of a child. This is in contrast to Scandinavian countries where significant proportions of parents take up the right to part-time work or leave at any one time (Land 2001).

New Deal for Lone Parents (NDLP)

As discussed in Chapter 1 and earlier in this chapter, the UK still has, of all European Union countries, the lowest level of participation in employment among lone mothers. Less than half of British lone mothers are in employment and some of these work for only a few hours a week, while remaining on out-of-work benefits. The welfare-to-work issues relating to lone parents in Britain are distinctive and form the background to NDLP.

NDLP provides a means for raising awareness and for promoting an understanding of employment opportunities and support from the state in terms of in-work benefits and help with childcare. It offers practical advice, including 'better-off' calculations for comparisons between out-of-work and in-work income, and can assist with the location of childcare services and, in some cases, short-term financial support for childcare. Most importantly, these forms of assistance are integrated with information and guidance about finding and getting jobs. Lone parents may have been isolated from the job market because of their social situation, so the significance of this aspect of NDLP should not be underestimated. Most lone parents are female and aged between 25 and 45, a group for which there are many and increasing job opportunities. Moreover, by reaching lone parent claimants at an early stage, NDLP can help to keep open a link to the job market at a time when it can otherwise be broken.

Financial and childcare advice, and practical job-search support, are likely to be the main drivers of NDLP's short-term impact. But NDLP also addresses some longer-term employment issues (Bryson *et al.* 1997). Low earnings capacity, resulting from a lack of educational qualifications and job training and experience, is a deep-seated problem for a large proportion of British lone parents, lowering the financial attractiveness of employment and prolonging reliance on in-work benefits. The National Minimum Wage, introduced in April 1999, is one method of tackling this problem. In the longer term, however, the issue requires educational and training investments to raise the 'human capital' of lone parents. NDLP provides advice and guidance to raise awareness of this issue and to offer pathways into continuing education and training provision but there is little practical/financial support for lone parents who wish to do further education or training.

While we have so far stressed the importance of economic and financial issues for lone parents, research has shown that this cannot be the whole story. For example, in comparing the British and Danish systems (White 2000, Pedersen *et al.* 2000), it becomes apparent that social attitudes and expectations towards employment must play a large part in the high participation rates of Danish lone mothers, since these are out of keeping with the extremely generous benefits offered there. Further, analysis of data on British lone mothers shows an important impact of attitudes on probabilities of employment, even after controlling for the 'objective' economic factors (Bryson *et al.* 1997). This point suggests that the overall impact of NDLP – including on the wider labour market – will depend on its success in changing attitudes and creating a climate of opinion in which employment is seen as the norm.

The NDLP was launched as a 'Phase One Prototype' in July 1997. Under the previous government, the 'lone parent caseworker' pilot had trialled some similar types of provision. The Phase One Prototype from 1997 onwards was voluntary and aimed to help lone parents on Income Support move into work, or towards work. Central to the new scheme were Personal Advisers who provided an integrated service of advice and support covering job search, advice on training, help in finding childcare services, advice and help on claiming benefits. All lone parents in the pilot areas on Income Support were eligible to take part in the scheme but it was particularly targeted at those with children aged over 5 and these lone parents were sent letters inviting them to see the Personal Adviser.

An evaluation of the prototype (Hales *et al.* 2000a, b) found that nearly a quarter of those invited to do so came forward for an interview. About one in five became 'full participants' in the prototype. Of these, 64 per cent said that they had benefited from the scheme. Four participants in five took a very favourable view of the Personal Advisers. In particular, participants appreciated the generally supportive qualities of the advisers (such as being friendly, outgoing, positive, enthusiastic, relaxed and confident) more than the practical assistance. This might have been important for lone parents lacking in self-confidence or perhaps concerned about whether or not they might be pressurised into looking for work. The prototype had a small positive effect on the number of lone parents moving off Income Support. After 18 months the number of lone parents on Income Support was estimated to be 3.3 per cent lower than it would have been in the absence of the programme. Most of those (80 per cent) who got jobs after participating in the prototype would have got these jobs anyway but one in five of the jobs were a more direct result of the scheme.

So far, the government has focused on getting lone parents *into* work, but given less attention to helping those in work to stay there. Improved maternity packages probably help and the government has made some progress here but more is needed. The same is true of family-friendly working practices in general. Similarly, it may be important to ensure that working parents are helped to remain in the labour force if and when they become lone parents. If more support were provided here (in terms of better maternity leave packages for single lone mothers and better parental leave schemes for widow/ers and those separated from partners), perhaps it would help such parents to stay in paid work.

Policies in other countries

Policies towards lone parents and employment have been changing in many countries. These changes have occurred in two main areas: the conditions under which lone parents are allowed to receive benefit (without having to work or be 'economically active') and the inclusion of lone parents in labour market programmes.

Table 6.4 (taken from Millar 2001) shows the conditions for receipt of benefit in five different countries. It shows that in all of these countries (except the USA), lone parents with pre-nursery school-age children can claim benefit without any requirement to be economically active. Once children reach primary school age, most countries have some activity requirements ranging from the requirement to attend work-related interviews (in Australia and the UK) to the requirement to be available for and actively seeking full-time work (in the Netherlands and Norway). France is the only country that relaxes activity requirements in the first year of lone parenthood (that is, for separated, divorced or widowed lone parents). In other countries, it is simply the age of the child/ren that matters.

Table 6.4 Activity requirements for lone parents as a condition of receiving financial support

Activity requirements	Youngest child is:		
	Pre-nursery/ pre-school	At primary school	At secondary school
None	Australia France Netherlands Norway UK		
Insertion*		France	France
Prepare for work: attend work-related interviews	UK (from 2002)	Australia UK	UK
Prepare for work: education/training		Norway Netherlands	Norway Netherlands
Seek part-time work	*(under discussion in the Netherlands)*	Netherlands	Netherlands
Seek full-time work	*(under discussion in the Netherlands)*	Netherlands Norway	Netherlands Norway
Take part in work or work-related activities	US	US	US Australia

* Insertion is based more on the concept of providing a right to work rather than an obligation to do so. It is therefore difficult to include under the other headings in this table.
Source: Millar (2001)

The UK and USA stand at opposite ends of the spectrum on activity requirements. The USA imposes a tough work requirement on lone parents when their babies are barely months old whereas the UK (at present) only requires lone parents to actively seek employment when their children have left school.

The other main policy approach for getting lone parents into employment concerns labour market programmes. Once again, these vary considerably across different countries (see Table 6.5, taken from Millar (2001)). Some are specifically designated for lone parents while others are more general labour market programmes. Some are compulsory to attend while others are not. Some involve a 'one-stop shop' and/or caseworker approach. Some have private sector involvement and/or the involvement of lone parent organisations. The focus of the different programmes also

Table 6.5 Labour market programmes for lone parents: summary

	Australia	Netherlands	Norway	UK	USA–Michigan
Programme name	JET	No separate title	OFO	NDLP	FIP
Designated lone parent programme	No	No	Yes	Yes	Yes
Compulsory to attend programme	No	Yes	No	No	Yes
One-stop shop	Yes	Being developed	No	Yes	Yes
Caseworker model	In part	Yes	No	Yes	Yes
Private sector contracted out provision	Yes	Yes	No	No	Yes
Self-help /lone parent organisation provision	No	No	Yes	No	No
Primary focus*	IA (WF)	HC	HC	IA (WF)	WF
Staged or phased approach	No	Yes	Yes	No	Yes
In-work mentoring available	No	No	No	Yes	Yes

* IA = Information and Advice; HC = Human Capital; WF = Work First.
Source: Millar (2001)

varies with some aiming mainly to provide information and advice while others are strictly 'work first' and others aim to build human capital skills.

A number of attempts have been made to evaluate the outcomes of these various programmes, with varying degrees of methodological rigour (see Millar 2001). Some of the most rigorous evaluations have taken place in the USA and these have shown that their programmes have had a positive effect on employment rates, in the context of a strong economy and in combination with other 'make work pay' policies. The most successful programme was found to be in Portland, Oregon. Its success has been attributed to the following factors:

- A strong employment orientation to the programme.
- High enforcement.
- Good job development and placement services.
- A relatively less disadvantaged welfare caseload.
- A good labour market with a relatively high minimum wage.

But these evaluations have equated 'success' with the number of lone parents finding paid work. Such 'success' might not lead to reductions in poverty as paid work is not necessarily a route out of poverty. Programmes that emphasise human capital may not be very successful in the short term in terms of increased employment but they may be more successful in the long term in terms of both increased employment and reduced poverty.

Millar (2001) draws a number of conclusions from her comparative analysis:

- Rules around requirements to work for lone parents are changing rapidly in many countries and the usual basis for requiring economic activity is the age of the child/ren.

- Compulsion is a complex concept in this field and should be discussed in relation to the nature of the compulsion, how it is operated, the context in which it is used and the type of sanctions employed.

- Local management and high levels of caseworker discretion are important features of many labour market programmes.

- Outcomes in terms of increased employment are relatively modest.

6.5 Should lone parents take paid work?

So far we have seen that British lone parents have relatively low levels of participation in the labour market. We have also reviewed government policies aimed at increasing this level. The policy debate is almost entirely framed in terms of the most effective and efficient mechanisms for raising levels of employment participation. We have also seen that in many countries, similar efforts are being made to get lone parents into paid work. But there has been relatively little debate (within government at least) about the goal of policy. We therefore take a step back to consider the arguments put for and against lone mothers participation in the labour market. Should lone parents go into paid work rather than work in the home as carers?

One of the main arguments in favour of lone parents taking paid work is that it makes their families better off financially while also providing a role model for their children to become paid workers. Kiernan (1996) found evidence that, in terms of long-term outcomes, children benefited from having a working lone mother. She found that daughters of working lone mothers were as likely to have attained qualifications or become young mothers as their contemporaries from couple families. Sons of working lone mothers had similar employment levels and dependency on welfare in adulthood as their contemporaries who had lived with two working parents in their teens. Research by Bryson *et al.* (1997) found that lone parents who took jobs and remained in them substantially reduced their families' levels of hardship. Longer periods on benefit increased hardship.

So there appears to be strong evidence that paid work improves living standards in the short term and outcomes for children in the long term. But this focus on the economic lives of lone mothers and their children fails to take into account their personal lives. Perhaps paid work makes them better off but contributes to more stress and is detrimental to the children. One of the main arguments against (lone) mothers working is that it is better, psychologically, for their children if mothers stay at home with them.

Tizard (1991) reviews the research evidence on the effects on children of mothers taking paid work. Of course, this research mainly looked at the effects on children in couples and so is not directly comparable to lone parents. Nevertheless it is highly informative. Tizard points out that, after the Second World War, research by Bowlby (1951) began to be used by those seeking to remove mothers from the world of paid work and put them back in the domestic sphere. Bowlby's classic study was used to argue that 'maternal deprivation' made it difficult for children to make relationships with other people. He argued that the crucial point in a child's life was between 6–7 months and 3 years of age. Bowlby's main area of interest was in children who were separated from their mothers when taken into long-term care. However, his research was seized upon by others and applied to mothers who had paid jobs. The World Health Organization (1951) stated that the use of day nurseries would cause 'permanent damage to the emotional health of a future generation'. And Bowlby himself went on to claim that 'to start nursery school much before the third birthday is for most children an undesirably stressful experience.'

Tizard's review of numerous studies, however, suggests that 'separation [of working mothers from their children] does not in itself cause harmful effects' (1991: p. 183). It seems that any adverse effects associated with separation of a pre-school-age child from a mother are due to the train of negative experiences that may accompany separation. These negative events include: the absence of other people to whom the child is attached; the child is in a strange environment; the child is passed from one person to another and no particular person takes on the 'mothering' role. Thus if a child is taken into a sub-standard form of institutional 'care' and does not become attached to other people, the child may suffer lasting damage. But if a child's mother (or main carer) goes out to work and the child is left with a caring adult to whom the child feels attached, then there will be no adverse consequences (apart, perhaps, from some initial distress at saying 'goodbye' temporarily).

Tizard also argues that formal childcare is not in itself psychologically damaging. She quotes the widespread use of childcare throughout history among the rich (in the form of nannies) and among the poor (in the form of childminders). She also quotes evidence that the model of the family in which the mother has sole care of a child is highly unusual in non-industrial societies. In general, studies in contemporary industrial societies have found little difference between children brought up by their mother only and those who have been cared for by others. In fact, some studies have found evidence that those who have been cared for by people other than their mothers have been less timid and more sociable towards unfamiliar people, and more willing to share with other children. Rather than seeing formal childcare as a second-best alternative for the care of children, perhaps society should see it more positively. Mothers and fathers are not necessarily good at caring for their children. Most parents have an instinctive love for their children but parenting skills are much less 'natural'. Formal childcare, with well-trained carers and appropriate resources, could provide a very positive environment within which to bring up children.

It is clear that there is little evidence to support Bowlby's claim that separation from a mother necessarily produces lasting psychological damage. Quite the opposite, children may benefit from mixing with other adults and children. Tizard (1991) concludes: 'For forty years in the West, women with young children who have chosen to go out to work outside their homes have been made to feel guilty and have been viewed as inadequate and selfish mothers.' While the current tide of opinion appears to be moving (slowly) against the condemnation of working mothers there is also perhaps a danger that non-working mothers (particularly lone mothers) will be made to feel guilty for not working outside the home.

Recent research by Ermisch and Francesconi (2001), however, seems to suggest that, if mothers work full-time before their children reach the age of 5, they will achieve less well in educational terms. However, the data for this study were drawn from children born between 1970 and 1981, a time when it was unusual for women with pre-school-age children to work full-time. There was no information in the dataset about the types of childcare used when mothers were at work and there was no information about the income levels of the families. These findings should therefore be treated with some caution.

Much of the research quoted has considered mothers regardless of whether they are with a partner or not. The arguments in relation to lone mothers are therefore likely to be slightly different. It could be argued that lone mothers (or indeed lone fathers) who are bereaved or who separate from a partner should spend extra time with children to see them through a difficult and sometimes traumatic process. Perhaps employment rights should include the right to time off for compassionate leave in such cases. And perhaps any requirement to work in the social security system should be waived for a certain period when bereavement or separation takes place. Lone parents may also face extra difficulties in combining paid work with unpaid work in the home. In couple families, there is always the possibility that unpaid work in the home might be shared between the couple to some extent. For lone parents, the complete 'double burden' has to be borne on a single pair of shoulders. Having said that, a woman who lives in a couple family and works full-time but receives no help from her partner has to do the washing and cleaning etc. for two adults where a lone parent has to do it only for one. There is a more room for negotiation in couples though this could mean more work or less work than for a lone parent. The stresses and strains for a lone parent are more predictable.

Very little of the debate about paid work and parenting has involved men. In the Netherlands there has been an attempt to encourage both men and women to work about 30 hours a week so that they can both share in childcare and domestic work (Knijn and van Wel 2001). This model would bring a form of equality that is rarely even dreamt of in Britain. This is not particularly an option for lone parent families, but non-resident fathers could be encouraged to play a large role in their children's lives. And if couples shared both paid work and caring work more equally, perhaps fewer would separate.

6.6 Summary

In Chapter 5 we had already touched on a number of issues relating to paid work as it is central to the government's strategy to reduce lone parent poverty and dependence on income support. This strategy places little value on the unpaid work in the home that most lone parents spend much of their time doing. Much of this unpaid work revolves around caring for children. In the past, 'mothering' work was valued in as much as it attracted considerable status for women. The state reinforced this by exempting lone parents on benefit from seeking work, as were the partners of unemployed men. From one point of view, such an approach is a positive one towards women as it enables them to carry out the 'mothering' work that they wish to do. From another point of view, it reinforces patriarchal assumptions that women's role is in the home. Not only does it lack any expectation that women might want to get paid work, it fails to provide them with any support, advice or training should they decide they do wish to get paid jobs. Men gain access to the wages from paid work and women remain dependent either on men (if they are in couples) or on the state (if they are lone parents).

The move towards encouraging lone parents to take paid work can therefore be seen from either of these perspectives. It can be seen as lowering the status of the unpaid 'mothering' work that women do or it could be seen as challenging women's confinement to the domestic sphere.

Very little of the debate about paid work and parenting has involved men. Their role in family life should be given attention alongside that of mothers.

Cultural views about work and motherhood are at least partly responsible for the rates of employment of lone parents. Only about two lone parents in five have paid jobs. About one in ten were looking for work in 1999 and a further one in ten might be said to be 'strongly attached' to the labour market. This leaves another two in five who have no immediate inclination to take a paid job.

The rate of employment of lone mothers in Britain is lower now than it was in the late 1970s. It is also much lower than in other European countries. In the past, lone mothers were more likely to have full-time work than all mothers but this has now been reversed. Why are the employment rates of lone parents low and why did they decline over the 1980s? Those lone parents who are keen to take paid work cite childcare as one of the most important barriers to work. Among those not so keen, the reasons given include the desire to take personal care of their children. One of the main reasons for the lowering employment rate appears to be the changing composition of lone parenthood – over the 1980s there was a big increase in the proportion of lone parents who were single lone mothers. These women had very young children and few qualifications and so were much less likely to get a paid job than other types of lone parent.

Turning to those in work, what kinds of jobs do they do? Lone parents who are in employment are mostly in low-paid, low-status jobs, often in the service sector. Their median hourly wages in 1999 were £4.40. Around six in ten were in jobs that could qualify them for Family Credit and about half of all working lone parents were receiving this benefit. About half of working lone parents were working 16–29 hours a week with the others working at least 30 hours a week.

Despite the difficulties, the government is keen to increase the numbers of lone parents in paid jobs. Its overall strategy has been described above in terms of 'making work pay' and 'welfare to work'. The New Deal for Lone Parents is currently a voluntary scheme that aims to encourage lone parents to think about employment. It provides help through a personal adviser. It appears to have been reasonably successful among those women who have come forward to participate in it. But a significant proportion of lone parents do not think that it is the right time for them to look for paid work – they place more importance in their caring responsibilities in the home.

Is the state right to encourage lone parents into paid jobs? The evidence suggests that paid work does improve living standards (though it does not necessarily take people out of poverty). And there is no strong evidence that children suffer as a result of mothers working. So it seems that the government is right to promote employment for lone parents but it should also find ways of ensuring that lone parents find work that pays them enough to give them and their children a reasonable standard of living.

chapter 7

Care and welfare of children

Much of this book has so far concentrated on lone parents. But, of course, there are also children in the lone parent family and this chapter considers the care and welfare of this group. The lone parent is not the only parent of their child/ren – in a sense this is obvious, but worth a reminder too. The non-resident parent may also be heavily involved in the care of the child/ren (widowhood excepted, of course). Other adults, both related and unrelated, may also play an important role here. This chapter addresses the role of non-resident parents (and others) in lone parent families. For widows there will be no non-resident parent; for most lone parents there will be only one non-resident parent, but for some lone parents there will be two (or more) non-resident parents of the dependent children. Non-resident parents may go on to have children of their own, in a new family, bringing with them new responsibilities and commitments.

Alongside the lone parent and the non-resident parent, the children in lone parent families sometimes receive childcare from others – either on an informal basis from grandparents or on a formal basis from paid childminders. The chapter will assess the use of such childcare. Finally, the chapter will consider the controversial area of the outcomes for children in lone mother families: are children's prospects worsened by living in a lone parent family?

7.1 Parental contact and care

Most children in lone parent families have a biological parent who lives away from them. Some do not because they live with a widowed lone parent. A few may have both parents living in the same home but leading independent lives. The role of non-resident parents in lone parent families has often been considered an issue in relation to child support (maintenance) but in this section of the book we consider the role of the non-resident parent in terms of contact and care for children. What role do non-resident parents play in the care of their children? What circumstances affect this?

Before assessing the role of the non-resident parent it is worth considering why it is that one parent (usually the mother) becomes the lone parent while the other parent (usually the father) becomes the non-resident parent. Many lone parent families are formed as a result of married couples separating and divorcing and so we need to consider the process of divorce that usually results in women becoming the parents with care. This outcome seems 'natural' to many people but is actually relatively new. In the nineteenth century, fathers (or more precisely, men married to the mothers of particular children) had absolute legal rights over those children. In effect, children were the property of the father. Women who separated or divorced from their husbands could quite easily be denied any future contact with their children. After 1839, divorced mothers who had not committed adultery could be allowed access and even legal custody to their children up to the age of 7 (subject to the court's discretion) (Maclean and Richards 1999). Women who had committed adultery had no rights to access. In 1873, the age of the children concerned was lifted to 16 and the adultery bar lifted. But it was not until the Guardianship Act of 1973 that married mothers had full equality with their husbands and the task of the courts was to make decisions based on the 'best interests of the child'. The child, however, was still considered as the property of his or her parents to be allocated to one or other (or perhaps both in the case of shared custody).

According to a survey carried out in 1984–85, children remained with their mothers immediately after their parents separated in the vast majority of divorce cases (Gregory and Foster 1990). In only 13 per cent of cases did children stay with their fathers and this was more likely if the children were older. When the courts intervened to grant care and control orders these usually reflected the arrangements made immediately after separation – only one in eight orders was granted to husbands. Custody orders were also generally made in favour of the wife – fewer than 10 per cent of such orders were sole orders in favour of the husband. It is difficult to find more up-to-date figures on this issue as custody orders are no longer made – parents are expected to arrange residence and contact arrangements for themselves. The courts only intervene if there is a dispute. Also, children might stay some of the time with one parent and some of the time with another. Also, they might live with one parent for part of the childhood and the other parent for another part of their childhood. Given the gendered nature of lone parenthood, however, it seems safe to assume that in the vast majority of cases, children remain with their mothers when their parents separate.

It seems therefore that the courts, and most couples, consider it to be in the best interests of their children to remain with their mothers. This is hardly surprising given that in contemporary culture motherhood is central to women's identity and to social expectations of womanhood. The consequence of this, however, is that lone parenthood is heavily gendered and it is women who both shoulder the burden and receive the rewards of sole parenthood much more often than men. It is interesting to speculate about how social policy might differ if men were the ones who more often took care of children after divorce.

About a quarter of lone parent families are the result of separation from a cohabiting relationship. And a further quarter are the result of births to non-cohabiting women. Until very recently, unmarried fathers had no rights over their children. Only married fathers had rights. Marriage and fatherhood has always gone hand-in-hand in law. This was partly because of the need to pass property down the patriarchal line and also because there was no reliable means, until quite recently, of proving biological parenthood. Today, paternity can be proved through DNA testing but the law still makes a fundamental distinction between married (or ex-married) fathers and unmarried fathers. Even if they are living with the child's mother, an unmarried father has no absolute legal right to give consent to their child undertaking medical treatment and unmarried fathers have no absolute legal right to care for their children even if the mother dies (Pickford 1999).

With the 1989 Children Act the terms 'custody' and 'access' were replaced with the more neutral terms 'residence' and 'contact'. In divorce cases, both (previously married) parents retain responsibility for their children and they are expected to come to their own agreement about residence and contact. As far as unmarried fathers' rights are concerned there have also been some changes recently. In 1990, Parental Responsibility Agreements and Orders were introduced. Agreements are made when both the mother and father wish to state that the father should be considered to have parental responsibility for his children. Orders are made when the parents cannot agree and the father applies to the court for an ordering conferring parental responsibility. These do not give unmarried fathers the same rights as married fathers but they are a step towards recognising the role of these fathers. Use of this legal provision, however, has been relatively limited. In 1996, there were 232,663 births to unmarried parents but only 3,000 agreements and 5,587 orders (Pickford 1999).

It is interesting that the law makes distinctions between married and unmarried fathers as far as 'parental responsibility' goes but the child support and social security systems make no such distinction. As we shall see in the next chapter, child support obligations fall squarely on the shoulders of biological parents regardless of marital status. So why is it that unmarried fathers are not deemed to have the same (non-financial) responsibility for their children as (ex-)married fathers? In the past, there has been concern that if parental responsibility were extended to all unmarried fathers some 'unmeritorious' fathers would be included. The idea behind this is that there might be some 'feckless fathers' or 'deadbeat dads' who cannot be treated as responsible. Such an idea seems derogatory to the hundreds of thousands of unmarried fathers created every year. And it also ignores the possibility that some (ex-)married fathers and even mothers might be 'unmeritorious' (Pickford 1999). It then begs various questions about what is considered to be 'unmeritorious', how such a label is applied, and by whom. Violent fathers would, no doubt, be included in this group and it would be difficult to argue that such fathers should have rights over their children (Hooper 1994).

One way of extending parental responsibility more widely, should we wish to do so, might be to grant it automatically to fathers who jointly register the birth. Joint registration implies that fathers are taking some share of responsibility for their children. Such a reform was, in fact, part of the Adoption and Children Act 2001. The government appears, here at least, to be valuing the role of fathers above the role of marriage.

Given the recent stance taken by the law on unmarried fatherhood it is therefore not surprising that, when a cohabitation breaks up, or when a single woman has a baby outside a cohabitation, the woman seems highly likely to take on the care of any children. There are no figures available on this, unfortunately, perhaps because it so widely assumed and practised, and because cohabitation is not officially recorded anywhere.

Once a lone parent family is created, a pattern of contact (or the lack of it) between the child and the non-resident parent will establish itself. In cases where a parent has been bereaved, there will obviously be no contact and there will also be no contact in some other cases. A survey of lone parents in 1999 (Marsh *et al.* 2001) found that 36 per cent of the children of lone parents had no contact at all with their father (see Table 7.1). This figure was much higher (61 per cent) for single, never-married lone parents. It was much lower (19 per cent) for those separated (but not divorced) from a husband. Where contact did occur it tended to

Table 7.1 Levels of contact between non-resident parents and their children

	All	Single, never- partnered	Divorced	Separated from marriage	Separated from cohabitation	All
	According to lone parents in 1999					According to absent fathers in 1995/6
Daily	6	5	2	9	7	} 47
Weekly	30	17	34	41	28	
Fortnightly	9	5	12	10	8	14
Monthly	7	3	9	8	6	7
Annual	9	4	12	9	9	10
Less often	4	5	4	4	5	18
No contact	36	61	28	19	37	3

Source: Marsh *et al.* (2001: Table 4.7); Bradshaw *et al.* (1999)

be quite frequent – weekly contact was most typical and more than 1 child in 20 had daily contact with their father.

These findings must be treated with some caution however. Bradshaw *et al.* (1999) carried out a survey of non-resident fathers and found much higher rates of contact (last column of Table 7.1). Only 3 per cent of their sample said that they never had contact with their children (compared with 36 per cent in the survey of lone parents). Much of this might be due to lone parents being more likely to say that the non-resident parent has 'no' contact if such contact is less frequent than once a year. But there may be other reasons for the different rates of reported contact (see Box 7.1).

The concept of 'contact' is a difficult one to operationalise and few research reports are explicit about what would count as 'contact' in their questionnaires. Some people might define 'contact' in physical terms such as meeting in person. Others might include direct though non-physical contact such as by telephone. Contact through indirect non-physical means such as by post or email might also be considered as contact by some but not necessarily by all. So perhaps if a non-resident father sends a birthday and Christmas card to his child every year he would count this as contact more than once a year but a lone parent and a child may take a different view.

Bradshaw *et al.* (1999) have looked into which factors affected contact between non-resident fathers and their children. They controlled

Box 7.1   Surveys of lone parents and surveys of non-resident fathers: why do they produce different findings on issues such as contact and maintenance?

We might expect that surveys of lone parents would produce similar findings to surveys of non-resident fathers on issues such as how many non-resident fathers keep in touch with their children and how many pay maintenance. However, there are often significant differences. Why is this?

● Surveys of non-resident fathers are not a perfect match for surveys of lone parents as some non-resident fathers will live apart from children who are now living in step-families rather than lone parent families. Also, some lone parents are men and their non-resident parent will be a mother but surveys of non-resident parents have so far been confined to fathers.

● Surveys are never perfectly representative of the population they are sampled from. Surveys of non-resident fathers face particular difficulties in this respect as they are based on asking a representative sample of men about whether or not they have fathered a child that no longer lives with them. Some men may not admit to an interviewer that they fall into this category, especially given the recent role of the CSA in trying to track down such fathers. Even if a man admits to being a non-resident father, he may not agree to giving a full interview about it. Those that do give interviews are perhaps more likely to be those who are in contact and paying maintenance. Some men may not even know that they have fathered such a child.

● People in surveys do not always tell 'the truth'. They may deliberately lie or they may simply see the world in different ways and so present a different version of 'the truth'. For example, lone parents may under-record the amount of maintenance they receive and non-resident parents may over-state it.

● Surveys often ask questions in slightly different ways making it difficult to compare the findings.

for a range of factors and found that the most important predictors of contact were:

● *The time it takes to visit.* If a non-resident father lived more than half an hour's journey time away, then they were less likely to have contact with their children.

- *New family composition.* If a non-resident father had a new partner and new children, then they were less likely to have contact with the children from a previous relationship.

- *Employment status.* Non-resident fathers in employment were more likely to have contact with their children than those not in work.

But Bradshaw *et al.* (1999) left out two important factors from their analysis. These were: relationship with the mother and the payment of maintenance. These important factors were left out because it was thought that they might be a *consequence* of levels of contact as well as a *predictor* of levels of contact. There is no doubt that these play a significant role in relation to contact but the precise nature of that role is complex.

Much emphasis is placed on the level and nature of contact between non-resident fathers and their children and yet few studies have looked into the relationships between *resident* fathers and their children. Many resident fathers could be working long hours and see little of their children. In theory, some non-resident fathers could be closer emotionally to their children than some resident fathers. For example, non-resident fathers might spend more time on their own with their children (that is, without the children's mother being present) and they might devote more 'quality time' with their children. Given their physical distance non-resident parents might put more effort into building up a close relationship with their child where some resident parents might take for granted these relationships.

James (1999) argues that it is not biology or even contact that is central to being a good parent. Research with children shows that they value a relationship in terms of feeling loved and valued. These feelings of being loved and cared for, especially for younger children, are most often described by them in terms of concrete social actions such as the provision of food or gifts, providing care when ill and accompanying them to different places. But it is the love and care behind such actions that are central. Children also wished to play a reciprocal part in the relationship, giving love and care back to their parents. The quality of the relationship is therefore not necessarily linked to the level of contact (although the two are likely to have some relationship). It is therefore important to bear these factors in mind when making assessments of the role of non-resident fathers.

Bradshaw *et al.* (1999) found that where non-resident fathers saw their children more than once a year, the nature of the contact usually involved visits from the children and overnight stays and so the opportunities to develop a close bond did exist. As well as looking at the nature of the relationship between children and non-resident parents it is also

Table 7.2 Nature of relationship between lone parent and non-resident parent, as reported by the lone parent in 1999

	All (%)	Divorced (%)	Separated from marriage (%)	Separated from cohabitation (%)	Single, never-partnered (%)
Very friendly	11	10	11	11	13
Quite friendly	30	28	35	31	23
Mixture	26	27	25	28	27
Not very friendly	11	13	13	9	14
Very unfriendly	21	23	16	21	25
No/too little contact	27	20	14	27	47

Source: Marsh *et al.* (2001: Table 4.7)

important to consider how well the lone parent gets on with the father of her children. According to a survey of lone parents in 1999 (Marsh *et al.* 2001), the nature of the relationships between the lone parents and the non-resident parent was mostly friendly but one lone parent in five reported that their relationship was 'very unfriendly' (see Table 7.2).

7.2 Non-parental childcare

Alongside parental care for children, grandparents often play an important role in lone parent families. Studies have shown the important role they play not only in providing childcare but also in providing financial and emotional support to lone parents (Kempson *et al.* 1994). Other more formal types of childcare, such as registered childminders, are also relied on by some lone mothers.

The issue of childcare has been an important one in the debate about the reasons for lone parents' low participation rates in employment (see Chapter 6). It is argued that childcare is not widely available to lone parents and even where it is available, it might be unaffordable. In the 1990s, the government introduced a number of policies in recognition of this issue. Before October 1994, lone parents received no help towards their childcare costs – they simply had to pay for childcare out of their income. This could substantially reduce financial incentives to work, making them worse off (or not much better off) in work than on benefit. A childcare disregard was therefore introduced such that, when applying for the in-work benefit, Family Credit, childcare costs (up to a particular maximum) would be deducted from their earnings before being assessed for financial support. This meant that the lone parent would generally, though not necessarily, receive more Family Credit if she was paying for childcare than if she was not (though the childcare spending would exceed any extra Family Credit awarded). In 1999, an allowance of £60 a week for one child or £100 a week for two or more children aged under 12 could be deducted from earnings for the purposes of assessing eligibility for Family Credit. Later in 1999 (October, to be precise), Family Credit was replaced by WFTC. This introduced greater financial support for childcare in two main ways. First, the age restriction was increased to 15 (or 16 for a disabled child). Second, childcare costs (or 70 per cent of them up to a limit) were added to the benefit payable rather than being offset against assessable income. This meant a considerable increase in the support available. Even so, the restrictions to only 'formal' types of childcare remained and this is likely to severely limit uptake of the disregard. By February 2000, about one lone parent in six on WFTC received help with the costs of childcare. The average amount spent on childcare was £48 (Inland Revenue 2000 WFTC statistics).

This section considers the types of childcare used by working lone parents and then addresses the issue of whether childcare is a barrier to employment for those lone parents (the majority) who are not currently in paid work.

In 1999, over two-thirds of working lone parents (those working 16 hours a week or more), had someone else to look after at least one of their children while they went out to work (Marsh *et al.* 2001). The rest, presumably, only worked when their children went to school or when they were old enough to look after themselves. Virtually all (98 per cent) of those with children under 11 used some form of childcare. In most cases (64 per cent) working lone parents had access to free childcare. This reflects the fact that most childcare is informal, supplied by grandparents or other relatives or friends (Ford 1996). For those who paid for their childcare, the average (median) cost per week in 1999 was £30 (Marsh *et al.* 2001). These working lone parents would, in theory, have been eligible to apply for the childcare disregard within Family Credit but this disregard was only available to those with children under the age of 11 and in formal types of childcare such as nurseries or registered childminders. As many as 85 per cent of all working lone parents used types of childcare that did not qualify them for the disregard.

Why is it that lone parents use childcare that cannot qualify for financial support? Are lone parents aware that the childcare disregard can give them financial help towards the cost of childcare? In 1994, when the disregard was introduced, and publicised widely, six in ten lone parents had heard that the government would provide 'help with childcare charges from social security'. According to Ford's qualitative study (Ford 1996), 'most' lone parents were aware of the disregard but they did not know enough about how it worked for it to alter their perceptions of financial incentives. Others were sure that it would not apply to them because their children were too old or because they had no plans to pay for formal childcare. So, according to Ford (1996), the childcare disregard appears to have had relatively limited impact for a number of reasons, including the following:

● Some lack of awareness of its existence.

● Some lack of knowledge about how it works.

● Restrictions on the age of children eligible – some lone parents wished to pay for childcare until their children are 13 years old but the disregard was available only up to the age of 11.

● Restrictions on the sources of childcare eligible – many lone parents preferred to employ grandparents or other informal childcarers and these would not be eligible for the disregard.

● General orientations to work/family among lone parents – some lone parents see childcare as their job and do not wish to use any other source of childcare (see below).

The issues of childcare availability and affordability have been highlighted in government policy but there is another important aspect of childcare that may affect a lone parent's ability to take up *and remain in* employment: reliability. Virtually all (98 per cent) of working lone parents said that their childcare was reliable (Marsh *et al.* 2001). Indeed, it is unlikely that they would have been able to sustain their jobs if their childcare was unreliable. Nevertheless, 61 per cent had made contingency plans for alternative childcare should their usual source be unavailable.

Among working lone parents, therefore, the majority use childcare that is free and reliable. What about non-employed lone parents? Is childcare a barrier to paid work? As mentioned in Chapter 6, the most common reason for not working given by non-employed lone parents was that they did not wish to spend more time away from their children (27 per cent) (Marsh *et al.* 2001). But almost a quarter said that difficulties affording childcare were a problem and 16 per cent said that the lack of available childcare was also an issue. Among those actually looking for work, the affordability and availability of childcare were the two most commonly mentioned barriers by far.

When asked what type of childcare they would prefer were they to take on paid work, non-employed lone parents were more likely to mention formal sources (such as registered childminders) than working lone parents (Ford 1996). One barrier to work might therefore be that non-employed lone parents have less access to informal and cheap (or free) sources than those in work.

In-depth interviews by Ford (1996) have explored the issue of child-care in greater detail. He argues that some, perhaps many, non-employed lone parents feel that it is *their* job to provide childcare and so do not wish to take a paid job and find (and perhaps pay) someone else to take over their childcare role. This takes us back to the discussions in Chapter 6 over orientations to work and family life. It also takes us back to the discussions about the outcomes for children of their parents working. Deepseated feelings about the negative outcomes of 'maternal deprivation' may influence lone parents' views and choices about the use of childcare. Other factors also affect views about the use of childcare such as 'legal status, media interest, social and private discourse, experience and prejudice' (Ford 1996). These factors will affect both whether or not childcare is used at all, and which particular types of childcare are called upon. For example, it may be deemed more acceptable for babies and very young children to be left in the care of a grandmother than to be put in a nursery. This may reflect a reluctance on the part of mothers to commodify love and care. In other words, they may have moral reservations about paying cash in return for someone to care for their child.

The issue of acceptability/suitability is therefore one that government needs to address if it is to succeed in significantly increasing the labour force participation of lone parents. But even if childcare were universally available and free, some, perhaps many, lone parents may still prefer to provide childcare themselves even if this means that they are financially worse off as a result. Of course, if a grandparent is willing and able to provide free and flexible childcare then perhaps this is a good thing. It is certainly a good thing for the lone parent but once again it involves people (usually women in the guise of grandmothers) giving their labour unpaid. It fails to recognise the importance of the caring work usually done by women.

The issue of quality also needs to be mentioned. Concern is often expressed about the quality of formal childcare provided by nurseries and childminders. While this is indeed an issue to be concerned about, it is often taken for granted that care provided by mothers (and other forms of informal care such as that provided by grandmothers) is of high quality. It could well be the case, however, that some types of formal childcare are of higher quality than informal types, though we need to think care-fully about what we would define as 'quality' here.

7.3 Outcomes for children

One of the most controversial areas in relation to lone parent families is the outcome for children. Many studies have tried to evaluate the effect of living in a lone parent family on children. Is lone parenthood detrimental to children? This question often divides people on political lines and relates strongly to debates about the 'death of the family'. Many on the right of the political spectrum argue that lone parenthood is an undesirable family state and one that has negative consequences for children. They argue that it should be discouraged and that policies should be aimed at encouraging people to get married before having children, and stay married afterwards, whatever the personal difficulties that may arise. Some on the left, and feminists in particular, argue that lone parent families do not necessarily cause difficulties for children. They tend to argue that any negative experiences for children in these families are the result of the material poverty they experience rather than any factor specific to the structure of lone parent families. Furthermore, 'staying together' may not always be a better option for the children, particularly in cases where there is violence and/or a high level of conflict.

Methodological difficulties measuring outcomes

Given the importance of this issue it is not surprising that there has been a great deal of research in this field. But there are great difficulties in carrying out such research and coming to strong, reliable conclusions. Much of the research has focused on the effects of divorce on children, as divorce has been perceived as a potential social problem since the 1970s. Research into the effects of single, never-married lone parenthood, for example, is less common. The research has tried to find out whether, other things being equal, lone parenthood has a detrimental effect on children. However, it is extremely difficult to keep 'other things equal' and compare lone parent families with otherwise similar couple families. A number of studies have used cohort surveys which have data on children from birth until well into adulthood (such as the National Survey of Children in the USA or the National Child Development Study in the UK). They then compare adults who, while children, went through parental separation and/or lone parenthood with adults who have had no such experiences. But those who have such experiences are much more likely to come from different and, in particular, poorer backgrounds and so it is difficult to control adequately for poverty (and other factors) and hence to be sure that any difference in outcome is due solely to the experience of parental separation and/or lone parenthood.

It is also difficult for research to take account of the fact that lone parenthood is usually a transitory state. It is therefore difficult to compare 'lone parent families' with 'couple families' because these two groups are not monolithic blocks but shifting groups. A couple family at one point in time will be a lone parent family at another point in time. Should researchers simply compare children who have always lived in a married couple family with children who have always lived in a lone parent family? But this latter case will not be typical of all children who have ever lived in a lone parent family. Another approach that, in theory at least, we might wish to take is to ask in relation to lone parents who have separated from a partner: 'would the children have been better off if the couple had not separated?' This is an impossible question to answer rigorously with empirical data as it is entirely hypothetical but it is the kind of question that we ultimately wish to know the answer to. Lone parenthood might be better for children than remaining in a family beset by arguments, anxiety and perhaps violence (see Chapter 2 for discussion about the extent of domestic violence).

Another issue for any research in this field is the type of outcome measures we are looking for. Much of the research looks at outcomes of divorce or lone parenthood for children after they reach adulthood, such as rates of unemployment, teenage pregnancy or lone parenthood and rates of imprisonment. It is therefore firmly situated in the discourse of 'children as the adults they will become'. Some research also looks at more immediate outcomes such as rates of truancy, levels of health and educational achievement. There has been relatively little research, however, that has talked directly to children about how they feel about being in a lone parent family and comparing similar children in couple families.

Finally, research must take into account the fact that the experience of divorce for children would have been very different in the 1950s compared with the 1960s, 1970s, 1980s, 1990s and after. As divorce becomes more widespread, it becomes less stigmatised and there are more support mechanisms available for parents and children. The same is true for the experience of growing up with a single never-married mother. To be born illegitimate in the 1950s would have caused great scandal (one reason for 'shotgun weddings' and forced adoptions). Today it is more widespread and attracts less (though still some) social disapproval. Research must therefore take into account the context within which these events and processes take place.

Box 7.2 sums up many of these methodological issues.

Box 7.2   Methodological difficulties measuring outcomes for children

1.   Lone parent families are different from couple families (for example in terms of higher poverty rates). It is therefore difficult to assert that any difference in outcome is due to differences in family structure rather than other factors such as poverty.

2.   Lone parenthood is a transitory state. Should we compare children who have always lived in a lone parent family with those who have always lived in a couple family? Or should we compare those who have *ever* lived in a lone parent family with those who have always lived in a couple family? A decision like this could dramatically affect the nature of the results from any research study. And we also need to consider that lone parenthood might affect children differently according to factors such as gender and age.

3.   The nub of the question is a hypothetical one: would children do better if their parents did not separate or if their mother had a partner before giving birth? Such hypotheticals are impossible to answer.

4.   Few studies have asked children directly for their views on this issue mostly, perhaps, because of ethical dilemmas in discussing such sensitive issues.

5.   Research must take into account the changing times. We can measure only adult outcomes on children who lived in lone parent families in the past. The experience of children living today in lone parent families is likely to be rather different. Evidence from the past cannot be used to predict the future in this area.

Research findings

Research in this field is, as we have seen, fraught with difficulties and dilemmas. Nevertheless it is vitally important. A number of researchers have reviewed the available (and sometimes conflicting) research evidence relating to the effects of divorce and/or lone parenthood on children. Furstenberg and Cherlin (1991) considered the effects of divorce on children in the USA and identified three important phases in the divorce process. The first phase could easily be overlooked by researchers and is the pre-separation phase. Furstenberg and Cherlin found evidence that children whose parents eventually divorced had exhibited behavioural problems well before separation occurred. In theory, such behavioural problems could have put strains on the marriage and contributed to the separation, but Furstenberg and Cherlin argued that conflict between the parents may have been the source of the children's problems prior to separation. This conclusion is supported by other evidence that children in intact families where there is a high level of conflict between the parents have similar (and sometimes worse) outcomes than children in families where divorce occurs. It is therefore the level of conflict between parents that causes difficulties for children.

Furstenberg and Cherlin did not claim that separation and divorce had no negative effects for children. On hearing of their parents' separation, research shows that children are usually upset. Some blame themselves for the separation, some are frightened and bewildered, and some are anxious and angry. The period immediately following the separation is the second important phase identified by Furstenberg and Cherlin. It has been termed the 'crisis period' by some researchers and it is a difficult time for both the parents and the children. Furstenberg and Cherlin (1991: p. 67) conclude that:

> almost all children are moderately or severely distressed when their parents separate and . . . most continue to experience confusion, sadness, or anger for a period of months or even years. Nevertheless, the most careful studies show a great deal of variation in the short-term reactions of children – even within the same family.

Age and gender account for some of this variation but researchers have so far been unable to explain all of it.

What about the long-term effects of divorce and lone parenthood? This is the third phase identified by Furstenberg and Cherlin who state that much less is known about this than about the second phase. Furstenberg and Cherlin point to a study by Peterson and Zill (1986) who found that, other things being equal, 34 per cent of parents who had separated or divorced said that their children had had behaviour or discipline problems at school resulting in a note or being asked to come in and talk to a teacher. The figure for parents in couple families was 20 per cent. This finding, like many other in this discussion, can be interpreted in two ways. We can argue that the percentage of parents from disrupted families who said that their children had behavioural problems was at least half again as large as the percentage of parents from couple families. This is a substantial difference. On the other hand, we could argue that two-thirds or 66 per cent of parents from disrupted families did not say that there were any behavioural problems. In other words, the rate of some problems might be more common in lone parents, but such problems are not, overall, commonly a 'lone parent problem'. We can therefore conclude that most children in lone parent families do not have such problems. Furstenberg and Cherlin refer to these two possible interpretations as the 'half-full and half-empty perspective' (p. 69) and they argue that both perspectives need to be kept in mind. In other words, most children in disrupted families do not suffer adversely in the long run but an important minority do. As Furstenberg and Cherlin conclude (1991: p. 70): 'there is no ineluctable path down which children of divorce progress. What becomes important then, is to identify the circumstances under which children seem to do well.'

Furstenberg and Cherlin identify a number of factors that appear to make a difference. These are:

- how well the custodial parent functions as a parent, which is itself related to the financial situation of the family;
- the degree of conflict between parents;
- maintenance of a close relationship with the non-resident parent.

While Furstenberg and Cherlin include the maintenance of a close relationship with the non-resident parent as an important factor affecting children's outcomes, they point out that there is much conflicting research on this point. They cite a number of studies that show no relationship between outcomes and the quantity/quality of contact between children and the non-resident parent. They admit that the evidence is 'puzzling' and 'mixed' but nevertheless believe that when parents are able to co-operate in childrearing after a divorce and where fathers maintain an active and supporting role, the children will benefit. The reason for lack of research evidence on this, they suggest, is that such families are probably highly unusual.

There has long been debate about the desirability of fathers keeping in touch with their children post-separation (Hooper 1994). At one time, it was thought best for children if their fathers made a clean break from them but in more recent times fathers are increasingly expected to maintain an active relationship with their children. In cases where fathers are violent, it is certainly not in the interests of children for contact to be maintained.

Burghes (1994) has also reviewed the available research in Britain on outcomes for children and found that there was some evidence that children fared worse in families where there had been 'family disruption'. But she concluded that:

> there is no single or straightforward relationship between family disruption, lone parenthood and outcomes for children . . . when families are disrupted the cause of that disruption may be more important in influencing outcomes, than is the new family structure in which children find themselves.   (p. 23)

Thus children in widowed lone parent families appear to have similar outcomes to children in couple families. It is therefore not the structure of the new (lone parent) family that might be detrimental to children but the way in which that lone parent family was formed. However, the act of parental separation must be seen as a process and, as in Furstenberg and Cherlin's review, there is evidence to suggest that much of the disparity in behaviour and educational achievement between children from lone parent families compared with couple families was found to exist before the separation took place. Burghes argues that this 'has increased interest in the influence that the **quality** of relationships within families have on children's development . . . a "bad" marriage may be worse than a "good" divorce' (1994: pp. 48–9).

Where family disruption does occur, Burghes argues that a number of factors help minimise the effects on children including:

- the mother's psychological well-being;
- the nature of the relationship between parents;
- continued contact with both parents;
- a secure and reasonable level of income;
- limiting the number of home and school moves.

A classic study by Cockett and Tripp (1994), known as the Exeter Family Study, analysed data comparing intact and 're-ordered' families. 'Intact' families were families where the biological parents had always lived (and were still living) with their children. 'Re-ordered' families were mostly lone parent families but a significant proportion were step-families. Children in these two family types were then matched depending on sex, age, mother's education, position in the family, type of school (state or independent) and social class group. The aim of this was to minimise the effect of these variables on outcomes. In-depth interviews were then carried out with parents and children in these matched groups. Cockett and Tripp to some extent dispute the general thrust of Burghes's argument that it is better for children if conflictual relationships are ended by separation and divorce. Cockett and Tripp claim (though provide no hard evidence) that an increasing number of separations occur through incompatibility or the wish by one partner to start a relationship with a new partner. Thus it is not outright conflict that appears to cause many separations but personal incompatibility – or less compatibility than is desired. While conflict is not necessarily the cause of separation it is, however, often a consequence, according to Cockett and Tripp. This perspective comes close to Giddens' idea that people today are keen to pursue 'pure relationships' rather than see themselves obliged to remain with a partner for life.

If this is the case, then it can cause difficulties for children. A particular problem for many children following separation is that they can no longer necessarily remain on the side-lines of conflict. They might now become the focal point of the conflict, for example over care and contact with both parents. 'Children also sometimes felt they had to suppress telling one parent about enjoyable times they had had with the other, or had actually been asked by one parent to keep something secret from their former partner' (Cockett and Tripp 1994: p. 58).

Rodgers and Pryor (1998) have also reviewed over 200 studies about the impact of divorce and separation on children. They concluded that children whose parents separate, when compared with children from intact families:

- tend to achieve less in socio-economic terms (work less, earn less);
- are at increased risk of behavioural problems such as aggression and delinquency;
- tend to perform less well in school and gain fewer educational qualifications;
- are more likely to be admitted to hospital and have health problems;
- are more likely to become sexually active at an early age, get pregnant, and give birth outside marriage;
- tend to be more depressed, and have higher levels of smoking, drinking and drug-taking during adolescence and adulthood.

Parental separation certainly appears to be very detrimental to children according to this list but Rodgers and Pryor do qualify their findings by reminding us that 'it cannot be assumed that parental separation is [the] underlying cause. The complexity of factors that impinge on a family before, during and after separation indicates a process rather than a single event, that merits careful examination' (p. 6).

Interestingly, Rodgers and Pryor also find evidence that children who live in step-families do less well than those in intact families and also less well than those in lone parent families. Thus, once again, it is not any particular family structure that is important (as step-families are more similar structurally to intact families than they are to lone parent families) but the dynamics and quality of family life. This research finding also suggests that the presence of two parents is not necessarily good for children's development (as children appear to fare worse in step-families than in lone parent families). These findings therefore suggest that it might be better for children in a lone parent family if their parent remains alone rather than forms a step-family.

Rodgers and Pryor do not find evidence to support widespread assumptions that the age at which children experience their parents' separation is, in itself, important. Nor do they conclude that boys are more adversely affected by parental separation than girls – although they do allow for the fact that girls and boys may exhibit distress in different ways. They do, however, find evidence to support an often-quoted fact that financial hardship and other socio-economic circumstances play an influential role in limiting children's educational achievements.

Some studies have asked children directly about their experiences of divorce and found that parents do not always tell their children of impending divorce but that children often pick up early clues and then look for further evidence (Mitchell 1984). This is because parents see their role as one of protecting their children. But, equally, children see their role as protecting their parents. Once they discover the truth about the impending divorce, children often hide their feelings so as not to upset their parents: 'some children had cried alone and deliberately out of sight of their parents whom they had not wanted to upset any further' (Mitchell 1984: p. 94). Just as parents had an ethic of care towards their children so too children had an ethic of care towards their parents. The findings from this study dispute the notion of children as passive beings or victims needing protection. They are active contributors to the child–parent relationship and just as keen to provide protection as receive it.

Cockett and Tripp (1994) found, perhaps not surprisingly, that children who had been in a violent couple family were very relieved when the parents separated. But children from these families nevertheless felt a mixture of feelings towards the non-resident parent, including sadness and anger. It seems that, in some cases, they would have preferred the violence to stop and the couple to remain together rather than the couple to separate. But they preferred their parents to separate rather than remain in a violent relationship. Children who have experienced violence between their parents at least understand why the relationship has ended. Children in other families do not always have such an understanding.

According to Cockett and Tripp (1994: p. 57) 'they are given little explanation at the time and inadequate arrangements are made for continuing contact with the parent who is leaving home. Children are left confused and bewildered, often hoping for a reconciliation for far longer than their parents imagine.'

Implications of the research

What conclusions do we draw from all this evidence? Should we argue for a return to the nuclear family of the 1950s? Should parents stay together 'for the sake of the children'? Should single women be discouraged from having babies outside a stable or married relationship? Or should we argue for giving more support to children who experience family disruption? Should we be promoting greater conciliation and mediation between parents both within relationships and after relationships have ended? These are highly complex and emotive questions.

The evidence suggests that it is not the fact of separation or living in a lone parent family that is, in itself, problematic for children. It is the factors usually associated with this that cause problems, most importantly lack of money and conflict between parents. Similarly, children suffer in couple relationships where there is lack of money and/or conflict between parents. The answer is to tackle these root causes of children's difficulties rather than to seek to promote one form of family structure over another.

Having said this, there is evidence that separation and divorce certainly cause short-term difficulties for children and may cause long-term difficulties, particularly if conflict goes unresolved or increases. Where the conflict within a relationship is overwhelming and unresolvable (perhaps including violence, alcohol or drug abuse) it is impossible to argue that the relationship should continue. However, at the other extreme (where there is no conflict but a degree of incompatibility), separation may increase the happiness of one, or both, partners but may cause short-term and perhaps long-term negative consequences for the children. In the past, the institution of marriage was a difficult one to escape from, even when the reality involved high levels of conflict and even violence. Today, people are more able to make individual lifestyle choices about marriage and sometimes there will be conflict between what is in the best interests of children and parents. Will the positive effects of separation/divorce be outweighed by the negative effects? Will separation be beneficial to some of the parties involved but not the others? Will it be highly beneficial to some but slightly detrimental to others? Or will it be slightly beneficial to some but highly detrimental to others? And should outcomes for children be weighted differently from outcomes for parents?

Research into relationship problems often highlights the role of better communication and mediation between partners but little is generally said about the way parents communicate with children. Research reviewed here suggests that children need more information about what is going on. Parents should beware the temptation to over-protect their children and should recognise the capacity children have to deal with difficult situations and provide support for parents as well as requiring support themselves.

The discussion so far has been dominated by the debate about the effects of separation or divorce. What about single, never-married lone parenthood? There has been much less research here because the increase in the number of single lone mothers is relatively recent. But we know that these families are often the poorest of all lone parents and, as we have seen, children suffer greatly owing to financial deprivation. We might also speculate that children in these families are less likely to experience parental conflict as they have never lived with two parents together. But there may be conflict with the non-resident parent in terms of contact or maintenance. If there is no contact at all there is likely to be no conflict but the children will then lack an adult male role model and a role model of a father. This may impact differently on sons and daughters. Many single, never-married lone mothers get together (and often marry) a partner within a few years of having a baby. The duration and quality of these relationships will therefore be key to the experiences and ultimate outcomes of their children.

7.4 Summary

Much of the debate about lone parenthood, including any discussion of employment, often ignores the children within these families. It also too often ignores the role of other people in the care of these children. For example non-resident parents are discussed at length in terms of child support but the state says little about the role of these people in terms of physical and emotional care for their children. This is because the state does not consider it appropriate to 'interfere' in private matters – material and financial welfare appear to be public issues in a way that physical and emotional welfare are not. Of course the state will get involved in extreme cases, where a child is under threat of harm from family members, but it does little to promote the well-being of children within families.

Non-resident parents in the UK are mostly men and this is because women tend to take on the main caring role when relationships break down. This relates back to heavily gendered notions of parenting which equate motherhood with care. In the past, however, mothers had few rights over access to their children following divorce (reflecting the patriarchal power of fathers). It was only as recently as 1973 that divorced mothers had equality with fathers and the courts began to make decisions in the 'best interests of the child'. Since then, most children have remained with their mothers. The 1989 Children Act was a major reform in this area, replacing the language of custody and access with residence and contact. In divorce cases both (previously married) parents retain responsibility for their children and they are expected to come to an agreement over residence and contact.

Unmarried fathers in the UK have relatively few rights in this area though they have been able, since 1990, to make a Parental Responsibility Agreement with the mother or apply for a Parental Responsibility Order if the mother will not co-operate. However, there has been very little up-take of such provisions. While the law in this field makes a significant distinction between married and unmarried fathers, no such distinction is made in the area of child support. As we shall see, biological parenthood is the only relevant factor as far as financial relationships are concerned.

Research with lone parents suggests a rather low level of contact between non-resident parents and children. According to one such survey about a third of children in lone parent families had lost all contact with their non-resident parents. A survey of non-resident fathers, however, paints a rather different picture with only 3 per cent of the fathers saying that they never had any contact with their children. The research suggests that a number of factors are related to contact: the time it takes to visit the children; the new family composition of the non-resident parent; and the employment status of the non-resident parent.

Biological parents are not the only people who look after children. Many working lone parents, especially with children under 11, use childcare while they are working. In most cases the childcare is 'informal' and unpaid, provided by family and friends.

The acceptability and flexibility of different forms of childcare are important issues. Many women feel it is more acceptable to leave their young children in the care of people they know and trust rather than to other people. Perhaps there is a feeling that 'care' and love should not be commodified – bought and sold. There may therefore be some general preference for unpaid informal care for 'ethical' reasons. These might also be combined with practical reasons as formal care may be less flexible than informal care. If a lone parent has to work different shifts, a formal childcarer or nursery may not be able to cover certain times. Perhaps a grandmother would be more flexible here.

Now we turn to a wider question concerning outcomes for children. Do children have better outcomes, worse outcomes or the same outcomes if they live in a lone parent family compared with a couple family? This is a crucial question in the debate over lone parenthood. Numerous studies have been carried out to answer this question but the methodological difficulties surrounding it are considerable. Despite these difficulties, a number of studies have addressed this issue. A number of conclusions have been reached:

- Poverty is the main cause of worse outcomes for children in lone parent families.

- It is parental conflict rather than parental separation/divorce that causes problems for children.

- The period immediately following parental separation is often a 'crisis' period for all involved. Children are not always helped by parents (however well intentioned) who try to shield them from what is going on.

- Some children do seem to have behavioural problems following parental separation but most do not.

- A 'good divorce' may be better than a 'bad marriage' but divorce sometimes increases the amount of conflict between the parents.

- Children in step-families may fare worse than children who remain in lone parent families.

All of this points to great complexity in unravelling the effects of parental separation/divorce on children.

Most of the research has investigated the effects of lone parent-hood through separation/divorce. There have been few studies focusing specifically on single lone parenthood. The methodological problems here are likely to be even greater as single lone parents are even poorer on average than all lone parents. So it would be very difficult to control for poverty.

The evidence suggests that lack of money and conflict between parents are the two key sources of problems for children. These can also cause problems for children in couple families and so it seems obvious that government should tackle these root causes of disadvantage rather than concerning itself with the particular family structure that children live in.

chapter 8

Non-resident parents
and child support

Chapter 7 looked at the role of non-resident parents in terms of residence, contact and care of their children. To some extent, the state is neutral about this role – little is done to encourage non-resident parents to have more access or provide more care for their children. But the state is far from neutral in terms of the financial relationship that non-resident parents are expected to have with their children. This chapter explores this relationship.

Child support is taken to mean the financial support that may be made between parents (or possibly other adults) and children, where the parent no longer lives with the child. It will therefore be relevant for many step-families, and not applicable in the case of widowed parents. However, it is in the context of high numbers of lone parents receiving means-tested benefits that maintenance is so often discussed. And it is lobby groups associated with lone parents and non-resident parents that have taken the greatest interest in policy developments such as the Child Support Act.

This chapter explores a number of areas related to child support. First, it considers the obligations that are legally owed between non-resident parents and their children. Next, it considers the reality of child support, who pays and why some do not. Finally, we review the role of the state in the child support system, focusing in particular on the Child Support Act 1991 and the changes to the child support system that it introduced.

8.1 Who should pay for children?

The question 'who should pay for children?' is part of a much broader debate relating to parental obligations and children's rights. When parents are living with their biological children these questions are rarely asked and the state says little about how much parents should spend on their children or the ways in which they might spend their money. Of course the state will intervene at the extremes, for example, if children are suffering neglect through having insufficient resources such as food, clothing and shelter. But generally the state will not get involved. Questions about parental obligations are raised only when the state is forced to play a role and this is generally when parents separate and/or divorce or when women have children outside cohabiting relationships.

Views differ about who should be financially responsible for children. Four main models are discussed here: biological parenthood, marital parenthood, social parenthood and state support. Each of these will be discussed in turn and are summarised in Table 8.1.

Biological parenthood

In recent years, biological parenthood has increasingly come to be viewed as the basis for child support. In 1990, Margaret Thatcher stated that: 'Parenthood is for life . . . legislation cannot make irresponsible parents responsible. But it can and must ensure that absent parents pay maintenance for their children' (*The Independent* 17 January 1990). This emphasis on biological parenthood as the basis for child support obligations has emerged for three main reasons. First, advances in technology in the form of DNA testing have removed almost all doubts over paternity, where paternity might be disputed. Second, it is increasingly argued, as noted just now, that biological parenthood brings with it certain moral and financial obligations. And third, the increasing dependence of lone parent families on the state has led to a call for biological parents (typically fathers) to pay more towards these families.

Biological parenthood is inextricably linked to the issue of responsible behaviour around conception. It has sometimes been thought that if parents are liable to financially support their children for all of their childhood they might take greater care to avoid accidental pregnancies. This moral aspect of biological parenthood is combined with a financial one – if biological parents have an unconditional obligation to support their children, then the cost of the state's role in supporting lone parents would be greatly reduced – assuming that parental obligation could be enforced.

But there are a number of problems involved in the emphasis on biological parenthood. For example, where parents form new step-families and perhaps then move on to yet another new step-family, the complex web of obligations based on biology becomes ever more tortuous. And today,

Table 8.1 The basis of child support obligations: four models

	How would it work?	Reasons put in favour	Reasons put against
Biological parenthood	All biological parents would be responsible for financial support of children until no longer dependent.	Might reduce 'irresponsible' sexual behaviour. Decrease cost of state support of lone parents and children.	Technology has complicated the issue. Creates complex family relationships where step-families are involved.
Marital parenthood	All married parents would be financially responsible both while married and if separate/divorce.	Recognises the importance of marriage.	Penalises those married. State has to pay for never-married lone parents.
Social parenthood	All parents living with children would be financially responsible for them until no longer dependent or no longer living in same household.	Simplifies family relationships where second/third families are involved. Recognises the importance of social parenthood.	State has to pay for lone parents. Might discourage lone parents from forming relationships and might encourage fathers to leave families.
State support	The state pays income to cover the costs of all children in all families regardless of structure and economic status.	Recognises the importance of children. Eradicates child poverty (if set at appropriate level). Removes the need to chase maintenance payments. Reduces conflict over maintenance between parents.	Expensive. Severs an important link between parents and children. Might encourage women to have more children.

with changes in fertility and conception methods (surrogacy, sperm donation, egg donation, cloning and so on), the biological basis of parenthood
becomes ever more disputable. If a couple who are unable to have children have a child using donor sperm, a donor egg and a surrogate's
womb, who are the child's biological parents? Is the woman who gives
birth a parent or is it merely the sperm and egg donors? This issue is becoming a very live one in the USA where children conceived using donor sperm
now have the right to find the identity of their biological father.

Perhaps the next step will be for such donor sperm fathers to be financially liable for their children? Take another example: if a married couple who have been trying to conceive a baby for many years eventually have a child through official IVF treatment (donor sperm) and then split up when the child is 5 years old, current British policy says that the 'social' father is financially responsible for the child rather than the biological father. So why are not all resident/social fathers responsible rather than biological fathers? Sperm donors may be a special case but they do lead us to question the absolute and unconditional nature of biological parenthood as a basis for child support.

Marital parenthood

Despite its problems, biological parenthood is the current basis of child support obligations in Britain but it is not the only possible basis on which child support obligations could depend. As we have seen, marital parenthood has historically been the basis of child support obligations and there are still many who would argue today that marriage forms the most appropriate unit in which to care for children. In theory, a system could be constructed in which all married parents would be financially responsible for any children both while married and if they separate or divorce. Basing child support obligations on marriage would recognise marriage as an important and distinctive institution but it might also appear to penalise people who marry and then separate if these people are pursued for child support while others who have never been married are not liable in such a way. It may therefore create some disincentives to marry. It would also leave the state liable to pay for large numbers of children – those born to single mothers and to couples who separate after cohabitation. The growth in cohabitation and in single lone parenthood means that it no longer seems feasible to base a system of child support on this principle.

Social parenthood

The third model rests on the principle of social parenthood as a possible basis for child support. This would be where parents currently living with children would be obliged to support them. This would recognise the importance of social parenthood and also simplify the nature of relationships between families where parents move on to form second or even third families. But lone parents would then have to remain dependent on state support unless they took up paid employment and there may also be some disincentives for men to stay in couples where they face relationship difficulties. There would be little disincentive to conceive children outside a relationship. There may also be some disincentives for lone parents to re-partner.

State support

The final model involves the state itself taking on full financial responsibility for children. For example, it could set Child Benefit at a rate that covered the cost of children. This would go to every child regardless of whether they were in a lone parent or couple family and whether or not they were in a rich or poor family. Such a scheme would, in effect, be a basic income for children. It would eradicate child poverty as long as it was set at a high enough level and parents spent the money on their children (and this is where parental responsibility would lie rather than in providing the income itself). It would remove the need for the state to secure child maintenance from non-resident parents. The scheme would be costly but the government does seem to be making some progress towards such a scheme with its proposed integrated child credit. Apart from the cost, such a scheme might be criticised as severing an important link between parents and children. But this could be characterised in a different way as removing an important element of power that parents wield over children. Such a scheme might encourage women to have more children either living alone or with a partner. This would increase the cost but would also increase the population of the country at a time when it is declining and the ageing population produces its own costs.

From marital parenthood to biological parenthood

As we have seen, marital parenthood was the chief basis of legal rights and responsibilities for children until the twentieth century. With the growth of lone parenthood from the 1970s onwards, legal parenthood became eclipsed by social parenthood and in the 1990s, attempts were made to focus more on the biological link between parent and child. Under the new model, the fact of biological parenthood is much more important than whether or not parents were married, and whether or not they lived together. To some extent, marriage is becoming a redundant legal concept in this field (Eekelaar 1997).

However, despite the relative unimportance of marriage in setting the legal framework governing parenthood, Maclean and Eekelaar (1997) maintain that parents keep in more regular contact with children if formerly married, rather than having previously cohabited or having been (to use their phrase) 'never together'. This they appear to attribute to the greater longevity of marriage compared with other types of relationship. However, there is still conflicting research evidence about whether marriage *is* more long-standing than other types of relationship once we control for factors such as the year the relationship started, age, class and so on. And Maclean and Eekelaar's empirical data probably do not contain enough long-term cohabitants to separately investigate the importance of duration compared with legal standing.

The following sections of this book will discuss views of child support in more detail but it is worth quoting here from a survey by Maclean and Eeklelaar (1997). They found that mothers were strongly attached to biological parenthood as the basis for financial support for children, whereas fathers placed greater importance on social parenthood. Related to this, fathers were more likely than mothers to think that the presence of any step-children should affect the amount of money he paid to his first family. And fathers were also more likely than mothers to think that any maintenance should be affected if the mother remarried. An Australian survey quoted by Maclean and Eekelaar (1997) also found strong support for biological parenthood but also some views that formerly married parents should have greater rights to shared parental responsibility than never-married parents. So biology was seen as important but marriage was not totally eclipsed by the biological link between parent and child.

8.2 Who does pay for children?

Current policy is based on compelling biological parents to pay for their children. Evidence, however, suggests that, in lone parent families, only a minority pay regular maintenance. This section will give details of who pays, and how much they pay.

Data from surveys of lone parents tend to have consistent messages – although, as we shall see, studies of absent parents tend to give a rather different picture (Bradshaw *et al.* 1999). Among lone parents (but excluding widows), about 30 per cent were receiving maintenance in 1993. A further 8 per cent had received maintenance in the past, but in 1993 were not doing so. A small proportion (4 per cent) had never received maintenance, despite having an agreement to do so (whether voluntarily or a court order), while the clear majority (57 per cent) were not receiving maintenance and did not have any agreement in place (Ford *et al.* 1995: p. 80). The 1999 survey apparently showed lower proportions of lone parent families receiving maintenance but this can be explained to some extent by the changes in procedures under the CSA (Marsh *et al.* 2001). These changes have led to more payments being collected directly by the CSA rather than going to lone parents. Thus lone parents are sometimes unaware whether the non-resident parent is paying any maintenance.

In 1993, maintenance was more commonly received by lone mothers who were divorced (43 per cent) or separated from a marriage (31 per cent), than among those never-married (23 per cent). Only ten per cent of lone fathers received maintenance (Marsh *et al.* 2001). These variations may be due to differences in the types of people in these categories (such as class and income differences) rather than differences related directly to marital status. For example, cohabiting couples tended to have lower incomes than the married.

The mean amount of maintenance being received in 1993 was around £32 per week, with half of recipients receiving £23 per week, or less. In 1999, the mean amount received was £54, with half receiving £40 (Marsh *et al.* 2001). One quarter of lone parents on Income Support received maintenance in 1993, compared with 39 per cent of non-recipients (mostly, those in paid work).

The most common reasons given by lone parents in 1999 to explain why they had not pursued maintenance were that they believed the ex-partner could not afford to pay (31 per cent) or because they did not want to have any contact with their ex-partner (27 per cent). A further one in six (16 per cent) did not know where their ex-partner was (Marsh *et al.* 2001).

So maintenance was much more likely to be received by lone parents in paid work, and the more they earned, the more likely they were to get maintenance as well. Half of those on moderate or high incomes were receiving maintenance payments in 1999 compared with about a third of those receiving Family Credit and only 16 per cent of those who were not in paid jobs. There could be a number of explanations for this. First of all, the children of poor lone parents (those on Income Support) are likely to have poor non-resident parents who cannot afford to pay much in maintenance. And even if these non-resident parents can afford to pay something they may see little incentive to do so as the CSA (and then the Treasury) would gain all the benefit. In 1999, lone parents on Income Support received no financial benefit from maintenance. There may also be a third explanation. Where lone parents on Income Support receive maintenance, they will have an incentive to take a paid job as they would then be able to keep some or all of the maintenance on top of their earnings.

These last two explanations seem slightly contradictory: the first implies that there is no advantage to receiving maintenance while on Income Support while the second implies the opposite. These apparently contradictory explanations can be resolved if we consider the variable employment opportunities of lone parents currently on Income Support. Those with few opportunities (perhaps those with few qualifications and young children) will see no benefit in receiving maintenance on Income Support because they do not gain financially from it immediately and cannot find a paid job in order to benefit from it at a later date. Those with good employment opportunities will not gain immediately from receiving maintenance while on Income Support but may then recognise that there is an incentive to take a paid job, and these women are, at some point, able to take advantage of that incentive.

While surveys of lone parents suggest that only about three in ten receive maintenance, a survey of non-resident parents paints a different picture. Bradshaw *et al.* (1999) found that 57 per cent of non-resident parents said that they were currently paying maintenance. This is much higher than the figure of 30 per cent reported consistently by lone parents. There are a number of possible reasons for this discrepancy (see Box 7.1 in Chapter 7), all of which are likely to play a part. It is nevertheless instructive to explore the survey of non-resident fathers further to see the types of non-resident parents who are more likely to pay than others.

Bradshaw *et al.* (1999) found that, other things being equal, non-resident parents who paid maintenance were more likely to be in employment and over 20 years of age when they first became a father. It was also more likely that the mother would not be receiving Income Support and that they would have contact with the mother. Payers were also more likely to have a formal maintenance agreement but also to provide informal financial support on top of the formal maintenance. Non-payers said that they were not paying maintenance because they could not afford it, often because they were unemployed. Those who had previously paid but were not currently doing so were most likely to say that they had stopped paying owing to unemployment.

Bradshaw *et al.* (1999) went on to construct an index of ability to pay maintenance. They found that 38 per cent of non-resident fathers had 'no paying potential' (those on Income Support or on very low incomes), 32 per cent had 'certain paying potential' (those in high incomes) and the remaining 30 per cent had 'possible' or 'probable' paying potential. Bradshaw *et al.* (1999) argue that there is little room for more non-resident fathers to pay maintenance as only 9 per cent of non-payers had 'certain paying potential'. But their definitions can be questioned as they themselves show that 16 per cent of current payers apparently have 'no paying potential'. Why is it that some non-resident fathers with 'no paying potential' do pay maintenance and some do not? Government policy no longer allows non-resident fathers to claim inability to afford maintenance as even those on Income Support will soon have to pay £5 per week regardless of their new family circumstances. Bradshaw *et al.* (1999) argue that if a non-resident parent lives with a new family on Income Support and his ex-partner is in employment or has re-partnered with someone on a reasonable income this reform will lead to redistribution away from poor children to children in families on middle or potentially even high incomes.

There therefore appears to be little social justice in this reform as it could mean redistribution from poor to non-poor. Proponents of the reform would argue, however, that the more fundamental principle is that biological parents have a lifelong and *unconditional* obligation to support their children financially. And in most cases the non-resident father is likely to have higher incomes than the family with children.

In qualitative work with non-resident fathers, Bradshaw *et al.* (1999) present a slightly different picture from their quantitative study. They interviewed three groups of men: willing payers; enforced payers; and non-payers. A key difference between these groups was not particularly their income or employment positions but the amount and nature of contact between them and their non-resident children. All of the willing payers, except for one, had contact with their children. Payment appeared to work as a guarantee of contact with the child by making the relationship with the mother much easier. These fathers felt a strong duty to pay for their children and in some cases this duty was fuelled by guilt as they felt responsible for the breakdown of the previous relationship. Enforced payers and non-payers generally felt victimised rather than guilty. The majority had no contact with their children and felt that the mothers gave little support and in some cases actively tried to destroy their relationships with their children. These fathers did not feel that there was a legitimate need for them to pay maintenance. This was either because they felt that their own needs (especially if they had a second family) were a priority or because they felt that their ex-partner did not need the money. Furthermore, they felt that any maintenance they paid would be squandered by the mothers, not benefiting their natural children.

In an attempt to reduce conflict from divorce, divorce law has moved away from notions of blame, guilt and fault but these notions are clearly still very powerful and affect people's behaviour, sometimes to the cost of children's happiness and well-being. This is certainly the case in the field of child support.

It is clear from all of this that the fathers saw the mothers as the people with whom they were negotiating maintenance, and mothers rather than children were the people who received the money directly. This explained why the same father might pay maintenance for a child from one relationship but not for a child from a different relationship. Any feelings of absolute obligation towards children were distorted by the individual relationships with the mothers. Payment of maintenance was a negotiated process based on certain normative guidelines such as 'balanced reciprocity' between the mother and father. If the mother facilitated or even merely allowed contact between the father and child then the father would be much more likely to reciprocate in terms of paying maintenance.

Biological parenthood was generally accepted by fathers as producing an obligation towards children but this was seen as conditional on certain other factors, most notably:

● the perceived relative financial needs of the non-resident parent and the parent with care;

● the amount of contact the non-resident parent had with the children;

● the nature of the relationship with the mother when the child was conceived (whether they married, living together, or in a more casual relationship);

● the way that the relationship ended (involving perceptions of who was to 'blame' for the ending);

● the nature of the current relationship between the non-resident parent and parent with care.

These research findings echo those of Burgoyne and Millar (1994) who found that fathers supported the *principle* of child support but saw it as an obligation conditional on certain factors such as ability to pay, contact with the child and the way the relationship with the mother had ended.

Some fathers were concerned that the money they paid was 'invisible' to their children and so would not be seen by their children as a symbol of love and affection. Thus fathers liked to be able to 'earmark' maintenance so that it was clear to all involved (not least the children) where the money was spent. Lewis (2000: p. 3) characterises the desire to make payments visible through 'earmarking' as a mechanism for retaining some degree of control over the money. And the gift of expensive items that the mother could not afford 'gives the father additional power and status'.

Lewis (2000) argues that the child support system tries to perpetuate the traditional gender roles of mothers and fathers even though they do not live together. Men are required to maintain the role of breadwinner but give up the traditional rewards. This leads to 'responsibility without power or status' (Lewis 2000: p. 4) and might explain the link between maintenance and contact that many non-resident parents tend to make.

According to Bradshaw *et al.* (1999), maintenance was seen by fathers in a number of symbolic ways, including:

- a symbol of love and affection;
- a compensation for past failings in relations with mothers and children;
- a substitute for 'not being there' for their children;
- a guarantee for contact by easing relations with the mother;
- a recognition of a child's entitlement;
- a recognition of the mother's entitlement as primary carer.

Children's views of child support

We know a little about how non-resident fathers feel about child support but what about children? Until recently there has been very little research directly with children about this, or indeed any other, issue. But a small-scale study by Clarke *et al.* (1996) interviewed 12 children aged between 10 and 17 living in lone parent families. The study aimed to explore both the children's own experiences and also their views of the general principles behind child support.

The children almost all saw biological fathers as having an unconditional obligation to provide support to their children. This absolutist view differed slightly from the views of a sample of mothers, including their own mothers (all of whom had been interviewed as part of a previous study). The mothers had felt that other factors affected the obligations of non-resident parents. Most notably, mothers felt that where a conception had been planned as part of a long-term relationship, there was a strong obligation on the father to maintain support. But if a conception had not been planned or not been part of a long-term relationship, there was less of an obligation. Children took a rather different view. They separated obligations for child support from other factors such as relationships between parents at conception or who ended the relationship.

The children also believed that fathers' obligations went beyond providing financial support. They thought that fathers should also provide other forms of concrete support to lone mothers, such as giving them a break from their caring responsibilities. They also identified maintaining contact as being a key parental responsibility but saw this as deriving from their rights as children rather than being linked to child support payments. This shows that the state's focus on financial responsibility obscures other important responsibilities attached to parenthood such as those relating to the level and quality of contact.

The views of children are rarely taken into account in the policy-making process. Unlike lone parents and non-resident parents they have not formed groups to lobby on their behalf. Little research has been carried out into their views and the research that it is available is on a very small scale.

8.3 Child support and the state

The low level of maintenance paid to lone mothers (and therefore the relatively high amount of benefit paid to this group) was perhaps the main factor leading to the introduction of the Child Support Act 1991. This Act laid down the framework with which to pursue non-resident fathers for maintenance. The Act and its implementation by the CSA have been widely attacked from a number of fronts. Non-resident parents have criticised the formula for calculating maintenance as being too inflexible and taking too much of their income. Lone mothers and their representatives publicise the fact that, initially at least, lone mothers on Income Support received no extra money if the non-resident parent paid maintenance. The Treasury took it all. And all sides criticised the CSA for pursuing the 'easy target' non-resident parents – those fathers who were already in contact with their children and perhaps paying some maintenance. Other non-resident fathers who had little to do with their children were not tackled first. As a result of these criticisms, reforms of the system have taken place and more are being implemented.

This section of the book reviews the system, or more accurately systems, of child support before 1991. It then considers the 1991 reforms and the chaos that ensued from their introduction. We also consider more recent reforms.

Child support systems before 1991

Prior to 1991, maintenance payments had been set, at quite low levels, by the courts. The 1974 Finer Report (Finer 1974) had found that fathers were not paying maintenance regularly but it concluded that there was little point in enforcing payments. This was for two reasons. First, it was often the case that men could not afford to pay the full amounts set because they had low incomes and sometimes had new families. Second, even if they did pay the full amount, these amounts were too low to make a significant difference to the living standards of lone parents and their children. Thus there seemed to be little reason to enforce payments. Partly as a response to the Finer Report and partly as a result of low resources due to increasing levels of unemployment, the Department of Social Security reduced the amount of effort put into chasing non-resident parents ('liable relatives') for maintenance. Previously the DSS liable relative officers could negotiate maintenance agreements outside the main court proceedings.

Over the 1980s, the number of divorces increased and the courts encouraged the view that there should be a 'clean break' settlement so that the parent with care retained any capital (such as the marital home) from the relationship and could then receive her on-going income from the state rather than the father. The explicit ethos here was a 'clean break' between the adults, not the parents and the children, although this distinction may have become blurred over time. The 1980s also saw a decline in the participation of lone mothers in the labour market. These factors combined to produce a phenomenal increase in expenditure on benefits for lone parents and this was the context for the 1991 Child Support Act.

But the Act was not solely inspired by financial considerations. There were also strong moral underpinnings to the reforms based on a return to Victorian morals and a desire to bolster the nuclear family. The Act did not just target divorced parents but also parents who had never married or had never even lived together. It was thought that if unmarried people were forced to pay for 'irresponsible behaviour' they might think twice before engaging in 'casual' sex without effective use of contraception. Better still, as far as the new Victorian moralists were concerned, they might only engage in sex within marriage and then remain married forever to the same person. As Lewis (2000: p. 2) argues: 'The logic of the legislation was that men should have only as many children as they could financially support, in other words, that men should fundamentally change the way in which they had come to assume they reproduce and move on.'

In 1990, the government produced the White Paper *Children Come First*. This set out its plans for reform of child support based on the idea that:

> Government cannot ensure that families stay together. But we can and must ensure that proper financial provision for children is made by their parents whenever it can be reasonably expected.
>
> Foreword to *Children Come First*
> (Department of Social Security 1990)

The government took the view that biological parenthood incurred certain obligations that remained with parents until their children grew up. These obligations were not conditional on changes to their relationship:

> Every child has a right to care from his or her parents. Parents generally have a legal and moral obligation to care for their children until the children are old enough to look after themselves. Obligations are unconditional and last throughout childhood no matter what the changes are to parents' relationships.
>
> <div align="right">Foreword to <i>Children Come First</i>
(Department of Social Security 1990)</div>

The 1991 Child Support Act

The Child Support Act introduced a large number of changes but many of these can be summarised into two key reforms:

1. Child maintenance was moved away from the courts and it became the responsibility (from 1993) of a new agency – the Child Support Agency (CSA).

2. Perhaps the main change was a movement towards a formula-based system of assessing maintenance. The formula itself was rather complex, involving a large number of pieces of separate information. The formula was also set so that awards of child maintenance would generally be rather higher than had been the case under the courts-based system. And they would be updated on a regular basis, to keep track with general increases in the cost of living (as tracked through levels of Income Support) and with changes in personal circumstances.

Both of these changes had been central to Australian reforms of child support that had been introduced in 1988/89 and echoed in changes in child support in the USA. Both the British and Australian reforms had been influenced by the need to cut public expenditure on benefits for lone parents. But, in the Australian system 'there was also a stated concern about child poverty which was absent from the British proposals', according to Millar and Whiteford (1993). The lack of concern for child poverty in the British system eventually led to particular criticisms of the reforms. But at the time, the Child Support Act received cross-party support and was also generally welcomed by pressure groups supporting lone parents. Some criticisms were made, however, when the reforms were being discussed. For example, the reforms proposed that the CSA would disregard any past settlements. This meant that existing agreements could be overturned and, in particular, any property or capital settlements could be ignored. If a divorcing couple had agreed a 'clean break settlement' (in which the mother received the house in return for waiving her rights to on-going maintenance), the CSA could disregard this agreement and order the father to begin paying maintenance. This seemed highly unfair to men who had given up their homes on the understanding that they would not have to pay any maintenance. Now they would be told to pay maintenance without any automatic right to reclaim their homes. The government, for many years, denied that this introduced any 'retrospection' in law.

There was also criticism from lone parents about the requirement of those on Income Support to comply with the CSA in providing information about the non-resident parent. It was argued that this could lead to violence against them if non-resident fathers were angry about being identified. It could also lead some fathers to demand rights to contact with children even if (in the mother's opinion) this would be harmful to the child (either emotionally or perhaps even physically). Some lone mothers attacked the very principle of the reforms, arguing that they should not be forced to depend on men they no longer had any (positive) relationship with.

While some criticisms were made of the proposed reforms it was only after the Act was implemented in 1993 that a storm of controversy engulfed the CSA. This was for two reasons. First of all, there were major problems with the way the CSA was administering the new system of child support. The CSA's computers could not cope with the new formula. The staff of the agency were inexperienced and untrained, often recruited from groups unused to such work. They did not initially file cases alphabetically – an example of bureaucratic madness leading to gross inefficiency. And they were overloaded with work as the CSA had been charged with taking on *all* existing cases (rather than taking on only new cases as the Australian system had when it was first introduced). The second reason for the controversy was the growing criticism of the system and the CSA from numerous groups, most vociferously, non-resident parents. The complexity of the formula had meant that people perhaps had not realised what impact it would have on them until they received an assessment. In some cases, fathers were faced with major increases in the amount they were expected to pay. Many thought this unfair or simply felt that they could not afford the extra amounts. They were then faced with an inadequate bureaucratic machine that did not reply to letters in a reasonable time, did not deal

---

Box 8.1   Criticisms of the child support reforms and their implementation in the early 1990s

- The new system disregarded previous settlements including 'clean break' arrangements.
- The new system went for 'easy targets' rather than parents who were avoiding their responsibilities.
- The new system took on all existing cases at once rather than just new cases or phasing in old cases.
- The formula was complex.
- The formula increased the amounts taken from non-resident fathers.
- Lone parents on income support were compelled to provide information about the non-resident parent.
- The CSA was inefficient and had poorly trained staff.
- The CSA's computer systems could not cope.
- The CSA's customer service was poor.

---

appropriately with telephone enquiries and therefore compounded people's dissatisfaction.

There was also criticism that the CSA had decided to target 'easy cases' – the cases where fathers were already paying something to their children rather than those cases where the fathers were paying nothing. This was seen as unfairly hitting responsible fathers and demanding more money from them rather than trying to make irresponsible fathers face their obligations. Where past settlements were overturned, this could lead to new or renewed tension between couples.

Non-resident fathers formed powerful and effective pressure groups (such as Families Need Fathers and Network Against the Child Support Act), partly through networking on the Internet. They gained the support of many newspapers who published the news that some fathers were taking their own lives as a result of the CSA's activity.

Barnes *et al.* (1998) argue that the policy ran into difficulties for at least four inter-related reasons:

1. Structural problems arising from what the policy set out to do.

2. Implementation difficulties because of the way it was introduced.

3. Frustration with the administration of the policy.

4. Failure of marketing to legitimise the policy aims.

They argue that some of the most crucial aspects of any reforms of child support include discussion of the amount fathers have to pay, fairness between families, supporting parental relationships, enforcement, improved administration and better marketing of the policy. Barnes *et al.* (1998) point out that consultation with a wide range of groups will be vital to the success of any future reforms in this field.

Reforming child support in the 1990s

Criticism of the system and the CSA became overwhelming and led to a new Act in 1995. This Act reformed the formula in various ways. It took account of some clean-break settlements and long travel distances between fathers and children. It also provided for 'departures' from the set formula. The result was lower average awards but still in the context of a complex formula.

In Bradshaw *et al.*'s (1999) study of non-resident fathers carried out in 1996, less than half of the non-resident fathers had had contact with the CSA and only just over half of these had had a final or interim assessment. The majority of fathers with a CSA assessment thought the amount demanded unfair most commonly because it did not take sufficient account of their living expenses. Six in ten thought that the assessment would have an impact on their living standards and just over half thought that the assessment would have a detrimental affect on their relationship with their ex-partner, their current partner or their non-resident children. A third thought it would reduce the informal payments or gifts that they currently gave to their non-resident children. There was also evidence that some fathers might be less likely to take a paid job or only take one that paid better wages than they would previously have considered.

The CSA carried out customer satisfaction surveys in 1994 and 1995. The 1995 survey found that 45 per cent of customers (including both non-resident parents and parents with care) were satisfied with the service they received (Speed and Kent 1996). The figure for non-resident parents (34 per cent) was much lower than that for parents with care (53 per cent). Levels of satisfaction fell far short of the Secretary of State's target of 65 per cent. Overall levels of satisfaction were calculated on the basis of answers to a number of different service-related issues such as: helpfulness and politeness of staff; nature of communications; speed of access to the service; speed of response and waiting time at the office; nature of the office facilities; the nature of the form (whether or not user-friendly and whether or not requiring reasonable information). The main issues leading to dissatisfaction with customer service in 1995 were:

- long periods of inactivity with no CSA-initiated communication with a customer;
- friendly, professional staff who were often unable to actually sort out the concern or query of the client;
- difficulties when telephoning offices;
- failure of the CSA to acknowledge complaints and reply to letters.

As we can see, the survey did not ask customers for their views about the *system* of child support, only about the manner in which it was delivered. Nevertheless, it is likely that views about the system affected people's views about the service.

A new survey is being carried out as this book is being written and it will be interesting to see if satisfaction levels have risen as a result of changes in the system and changes in the way it is delivered.

The 1995 reforms made some improvements to the system but criticism remained and in 1999 a new government produced a White Paper on child support, *A New Contract for Welfare: Children's Rights and Parents' Responsibilities* following on from the earlier Green Paper (Department of Social Security 1998). The reforms will greatly simplify the formula so that non-resident parents will be required to pay 15 per cent of their wages for a single child, rising to 20 per cent for two and 25 per cent for three or more. Those on Income Support (who have been exempt from paying any maintenance so far) will now be required to pay up to £5 a week in child support. More maintenance will go direct to lone parents rather than being taken by the Treasury. Lone parents on income support will receive the first £10 of maintenance and those on WFTC will receive it all without losing any social security benefits. Alistair Darling, Secretary of State for Social Security summarised the aims of the reform:

> We're making it far easier for fathers to support their children, but we're being far tougher on those who won't.
>
> (DSS press release, 1 December 1999)

These tough measures include a 'one strike and you're out' ruling, where non-resident fathers who miss even a single payment of maintenance will see the money owed to their families taken directly from their salary (if they are in work, that is!). Fathers who deliberately try to evade the CSA will also face fines of up to £1,000.

The simplification of the formula is generally seen as an improvement but some critics have argued that the government has merely bowed to pressure from non-resident fathers to reduce the amount they have to pay. And there has been criticism of the plan to take money from non-resident parents on Income Support. Income Support is a minimum safety net benefit and any money taken from it drags people further down below the poverty line. If these people have new families, then the children in these families will no doubt suffer along with the non-resident father. The new tough measures against non-payment will win support only if the overall system seems fair, and this is open to question. The state sees child support as an unconditional obligation of biological parenthood. This is not how the parents involved (at least not all of them) tend to see it.

The White Paper (House of Commons 1999) does note the link between maintenance and contact, stating that: 'it is clearly important for successful child support arrangements that contact is settled to the satisfaction of both parents' but it makes little reference to how this might be achieved. Child support regimes in many other countries, for example, do deal with maintenance and contact together (Corden 1999). Skinner and Bradshaw (2000: p. 7) argue that 'there is no need to re-enforce parental obligations – they exist and are accepted already. But there is a need to facilitate them through an increased understanding of the emotional and moral turmoil that follows in the wake of family separation.' One way forward might be to build on the Lord Chancellor's department's experiments with mediation services. But Lewis (2000) argues that there is a more fundamental issue in terms of the way men see their role as fathers. The breadwinning role is well-established and is firmly intertwined with their role as carers. Lewis argues that it is important for men to distinguish between these two roles so that they might pay even if they do not wish to provide social or emotional 'care' and they might provide social or emotional 'care' even if they are unable to pay. The state has focused heavily on the breadwinning side of fathering and paid little attention to the caring side.

Learning lessons from other countries

We have already seen that the British system borrowed certain elements from the Australian reforms of the late 1980s. The British system also drew on the experience of the system in Wisconsin in the USA. Corden (1999) has reviewed child support schemes in Europe to consider what makes some child support systems work well. Before reviewing her findings, it is worth considering the more fundamental question of what criteria should be used to judge whether or not a child support system is working well (see Box 8.2 for Corden's criteria). Corden identifies five groups of people who need to be considered: children; parents in general and their advisers;

> **Box 8.2   Summary of Corden's (1999) list of criteria for judging whether a child support system is working well**
>
> **For children**, if:
>
> - it delivers a regular payment towards the needs of all entitled children;
> - it does not harm their relationship with non-resident parents.
>
> **For parents in general and their advisers**, if:
>
> - it is transparent and comprehensible;
> - assessments can be made speedily;
> - it is responsive to significant changes in circumstances.
>
> **For parents with care (including lone parents)**, if:
>
> - it does not discourage paid work.
>
> **For non-resident parents**, if:
>
> - payments are affordable.
>
> **For tax-payers**, if:
>
> - it does not does not discourage paid work or encourage fraud;
> - administration is efficient and inexpensive;
> - there is minimal non-payment by liable parents.

parents with care (including lone parents); non-resident parents; and tax-payers. She then lists various factors pertinent to each group. While this list does not necessarily provide a full list of all criteria that might be deemed appropriate it does at least cause us to consider the criteria in more detail than politicians and policy-makers have perhaps hitherto done. Note that the list says nothing about the level of payment. And the interests of each of the five groups identified may be antagonistic, particularly when it comes to the level of payment.

Following on from her criteria, Corden (1999: p. 55) argues that the child support system in Denmark stands out 'without major problems or negative outcomes for any particular groups'. This scheme's success is explained by a number of factors such as its length of establishment, the simplicity of the scheme and its local administration. Payments are set at a reasonably low level and (perhaps as a result) there is a relatively high level of compliance. The low level of payments is not a particular issue for lone parents or tax-payers because lone parents in Denmark have much higher rates of participation in the labour market compared with those in Britain. This is partly due to cultural expectations that mothers should work and also to the provision of high-quality public services including child care. Those not in paid work receive relatively generous social security payments. In Nordic countries generally there is an emphasis on the rights of children to parental support or equivalent support from the state to maintain a decent standard of living.

Some European countries seem to have experienced problems where high liabilities for maintenance cause disincentives to work among non-resident parents. However, there is very little strong empirical evidence of this effect. The Austrian system has an advanced maintenance scheme which is relatively generous in the level and availability of payments but it has proved costly and difficult to recover the money owed. The Belgium scheme appears to work successfully as it is efficient and relatively inexpensive to run but it is also a less 'ambitious' scheme than others.

So far, it might seem that Britain was unusual in having severe problems with its system of child support but France and Germany have also faced difficulties. In Germany, there have recently been changes in legislation to reduce the complexity of procedures and increase compliance but these changes have been criticised as sacrificing the needs of the child to the needs of the non-resident parent. In France there is much discretion over assessment and this leads to the charge of unfairness in the system. The debate over the pros and cons of discretion versus rules is a complex one. Unfairness can be a feature of rules-based systems (as the initial child support scheme in Britain was criticised as being) as well as a feature of discretion-based systems (as in France). In France, there is also a significant problem of non-compliance.

In all countries except Denmark the affordability of payments is seen as a problem for some non-resident parents. This is argued to reflect real economic hardship facing some people in this group. For example, levels of payment are set high in Germany and are maintained through periods of unemployment, causing further financial difficulties for some parents. As Corden concludes (1999: p. 57): 'one person's income and resources does [sic] not stretch to two households.'

8.4 Summary

The state is fairly neutral about the role of non-resident parents as far as contact and care are concerned – parents are generally left to themselves to make arrangements on this. But the state is far from neutral about financial support for children. The state requires and enforces (in theory at least) a biological basis to child support. Biological parents have an unconditional obligation to support their children financially. This is not, however, the only possible framework on which child support could be based. In the past, marriage was the key to child support obligations. Men had rights over the children borne by their wives. With the growth in illegitimacy, cohabitation and divorce, the link between marriage and parenthood has declined and the best interests of the child have overtaken the patriarchal rights of men. But the obligations of fathers (albeit based on biology rather than marriage) remain.

The biological basis of child support can cause major complications where people move in and out of different family types. Should the state force ex-families to retain financial links once the bonds of co-residence and perhaps love and affection have disappeared? Will such obligations cause conflict between parents and thus be detrimental to children? Another framework for child support is social parenthood. This would mean that parents who live with their children would be financially re-sponsible for them whether or not they are married and whether or not they are the biological parents. Such a scheme would provide status for social parenthood at the cost of biological and marital parenthood. It would be costly in that the state would have to pay for lone parent families (but it does so mostly now due to low rates of maintenance payments). It may also produce disincentives for men to live with their partners and children.

Whatever the pros and cons of different frameworks, the current frame-work in Britain is clear: unconditional biological parenthood is the basis for child support. But research shows us that, according to lone parents, only a minority (about 30 per cent) of non-resident parents are paying child support to them. Surveys of non-resident fathers report higher figures of maintenance payment but it is unlikely that a majority of lone parents are receiving any maintenance. Single, never-married lone mothers are least likely to receive maintenance of all lone parent types. Of those receiving maintenance, a typical payment is £40 a week.

Why do so few non-resident parents pay maintenance? One way of approaching this question is to consider the types of non-resident par-ents who do pay. Payers are more likely to be in employment and be at least in their 20s when they became fathers. They are more likely to have contact with the mother and for her not to be on income support. Another factor relates to whether the non-resident parent has formed a new family or not. If they have new children to care for and support, they usually feel less obligation towards children from a previous relationship.

The 1991 Child Support Act moved child support away from the courts and DSS liable relative officers to a new agency – the Child Support Agency. It also introduced a formula-based method of assessing maintenance. The introduction of the reforms was a fiasco and the 1990s saw growing campaigns against the reforms; a number of further reforms were introduced. In 1999, a new government proposed to simplify the formula (and simplify it in such a way that it would generally reduce the amount non-resident parents were expected to pay). On the other hand, there was a new stipulation that non-resident parents on income support would have to pay up to £5 a week per child. Prior to this they had not been liable for payments. These reforms seem, therefore, to have softened the regime for richer fathers (who will probably have less to pay, unless at the very top end) but has hardened it for poorer fathers (who will now have to pay more if they are on income support). The government is also cracking down more on non-payers with tougher sanctions. The situation for lone parents on income support has improved as they will soon be able to keep some of the maintenance paid by their non-resident parents.

chapter 9

Health, housing and hardship

Lone parents (and their children) have relatively poor levels of health and relatively high levels of disability. They also live in poor housing. These factors, combined with their low levels of income, contribute to making this group among the most multipally-disadvantaged in the country. For some lone parents, the high incidence of such problems will be partly responsible for their poverty – perhaps poor health or disability contributed to marriage breakdown or resulted in them losing paid work. For some, poverty itself might be responsible for poor health and poor housing. For many, these problems will exacerbate the difficulties of living on a low income.

9.1 Sickness and disability

There have been few studies focusing on lone parenthood and sickness/disability yet surveys show that lone parents suffer poor levels of health and high levels of disability. There are a number of ways in which health and illness might be measured. For example, we can simply ask people to rate their health on a scale from very good to very poor. Or we can ask people whether they have a long-term illness or disability. In their 1999 survey Marsh *et al.* (2001) found that over half (54 per cent) of all lone parents reported good health while 30 per cent said that their health was fairly good and 16 per cent said that their health was poor. Health was strongly related to employment status. Three-quarters of those on high incomes or in self-employment had good health compared with less than half of those not in paid work. The relationship between work and illness/disability is an interesting one. Perhaps some workers became ill or disabled and had to give up their jobs. Or perhaps illness and disability make it difficult for lone parents to get jobs. Or perhaps being jobless causes some illnesses, particularly those relating to stress and depression.

Interestingly, there was little difference in health between the different types of lone parent – single lone parents had similar states of health to separated or divorced lone parents.

Another way of looking at sickness or disability is to find out what proportion of lone parents have long-standing health problems. Three lone parents in ten said that they had at least one long-standing health problem (Marsh *et al.* 2001). Once again, this was related to work status with non-workers more likely to have such problems. A study by Ford *et al.* (1998) categorised the types of conditions affecting lone parents in 1995. Thirty per cent of those with a long-standing condition had musculo-skeletal problems (back problems, arthritis), 17 per cent had respiratory problems (bronchitis, asthma), 14 per cent had mental disorders (depression, anxiety) and 11 per cent had problems with their nervous system/sense organs (epilepsy, strokes, MS).

Not only do a substantial minority of lone parents have poor health and/or long-standing health problems, they are also quite likely to have children with health problems. One-third of lone parents had at least one child with a long-term illness or disability (Marsh *et al.* 2001). This seemed to have an impact on their capacity to work as those lone parents with sick or disabled children were less likely to be in paid work.

As well as caring for their own (sometimes sick or disabled) children, lone parents also have to care for other people in some cases. About one in ten cared for someone other than their children because of illness or disability.

Box 9.1   Lone parents and sickness/disability (Marsh *et al.* 2001)

- About one in six lone parents say they have poor health.
- Three in ten lone parents have a long-standing health problem.
- One-third of lone parents have at least one child with a long-term illness or disability.
- One in ten lone parents care for another person because of illness or disability.
- Illness and disability are related to work status.

The study by Ford *et al.* (1998) looked at trends in health status and found evidence of a worrying trend towards worse health among a panel of lone parent families. In 1991, only one in seven (15 per cent) said that they had a long-standing illness. This rose to one in five in 1993, one in four (25 per cent) in 1994 and nearly three in ten (29 per cent) in 1995. More than half (57 per cent) of lone parents never reported a long-standing illness between 1991 and 1995 ('healthy throughout') but 7 per cent always reported such an illness. Among others, some saw health improve and some saw health decline. There was a clear link between health and employment status. Half of those who were unhealthy throughout or became unhealthy, never worked over the period of study. Some of this trend was probably due to the general ageing of the panel.

The study went on to look at changes in children's health and found that in 4 per cent of households, there was at least one child with a long-term illness at each study point. In two-thirds of households all children remained healthy throughout the study period. About three in ten had some experience of children with a long-term illness. Nearly 70 per cent of the reported health conditions of the first or only ill child in the household were respiratory problems (such as asthma). The second most common type of condition was nervous disorders (epilepsy). Households with 'ever-ill' children were slightly less likely to be in employment. Policy emphasis on employment may not be so appropriate for those incapable of work or with limitations or with responsibility to care for a child (Ford *et al.* 1998).

Taking adult and child health together, only four households in ten remained free of long-term ill health from 1991 to 1995. In 1991, a quarter of households had a member with a long-standing medical condition. By 1995, this figure had nearly doubled to 45 per cent. In 12 per cent of households in 1995, both the parent and one or more children had a long-term condition (Ford *et al.* 1998).

The poor health of lone parents should be placed in context of the more general links between health and poverty (Blackburn 1991, Acheson 1998). Poverty appears to cause poor health but why is this the case? One set of explanations lies in the knowledge, attitudes and lifestyle of the poor themselves. It is argued that they know too little about how to keep healthy and they squander their money on inappropriate goods such as cigarettes. The smoking issue is one that particularly relates to lone parents. In 1991, more than half of all lone parents smoked (55 per cent). This was a much higher rate than that for all women (30 per cent) but it was also much higher than for women in low-income couples (38 per cent). Among lone parents on income support who smoked, the gross cost was £9.20

a week, about 15 per cent of their disposable income (Marsh and McKay 1994).

According to Marsh and McKay (1994: p. 79) this had a detrimental impact on their material welfare: 'hardship increased sharply as smoking increased.' Lone parents themselves say that they go without other things to protect their children from the impact of their spending on cigarettes but the evidence shows that, despite lone parents' best intentions, children are affected: lone parents who smoke are less likely to have essential items for their children compared with those who do not smoke. Marsh and McKay (1994) concluded that smoking was by no means the only cause of their hardship but it was an additional one.

So why do lone parents continue to smoke? One reason sometimes put forward is that it relieves the stress they suffer from. Marsh and McKay (1994) argue that people who are successful at stopping smoking are those with optimism for the future. Lone parents generally do not feel optimistic and tend to suffer from anxiety and depression. This makes it very difficult for them to stop smoking. Dorsett and Marsh (1998: p. 122) argue that 'Lone parents smoke because cigarettes provide an affordable palliative for the stress of their everyday lives. This stress is the result of the disadvantage that lone parents face as one of the most marginalised groups in society.'

Thus there is a 'malign spiral' that locks lone parents into smoking, with links between smoking, morale, pessimism, poor health and even the reduced health of their children. Continuing hardship blocks their route out of smoking: 'Lone mothers remain trapped both in poverty and smoking' (Dorsett and Marsh 1998: p. 125). Dorsett and Marsh argue that the government should develop 'Welfare-to-Health' policies as well as Welfare-to-Work. Lone parents who smoke pay almost £300 million a year back to the Treasury – 17 per cent of their share of income support. Dorsett and Marsh (1998) argue that we need to use some of this money to tackle the problem and its underlying causes through more 'joined-up government'.

Apart from the issue of smoking, there is little evidence that the poor health of lone parents and their children can be attributed to lack of knowledge or particular lifestyle choices. Blackburn (1991: p. 154) argues that there is little evidence for this view: 'low levels of health knowledge, undesirable health attitudes and health orientations are not responsible for poor health among families in poverty.' She points out that poor families have similar levels of knowledge to other families and so knowledge cannot be the explanation for their poorer health. A range of studies (see Kempson 1996 for a review) have also shown that women in poor families are very careful in their budgeting and do not squander their money. The research shows that women generally know about healthy eating but find that certain healthy foods, including fresh fruit, are very expensive and it is very wasteful to buy healthy foods if children refuse to eat them. Biscuits and cakes may not be very healthy but they are high in calories and cheap and children will eat them (Kempson *et al.* 1994). Dowler and Calvert (1995) report that food is the most flexible item in a weekly budget and so it is often cut back to pay for other less flexible items such as rent and utility bills.

Many lone parents face an impossible task in stretching out inadequate income to make ends meet. Studies suggest that they make every effort to save their children from deprivation by cutting back on things for themselves: 'women appear to mitigate the effect of poverty on other family members by cutting down on their own consumption and expenditure' (Blackburn 1991: p. 155). This could have a negative impact on their own health, particularly if prolonged.

If knowledge, attitudes and lifestyle cannot adequately explain the links between poverty and poor health, what can? The explanation lies in the socio-economic conditions of poor families. Poor housing, poor diet, unsafe environments and lack of access to health and social facilities are all a direct result of inadequate material resources. Poor families cannot afford to live in high-quality housing. Houses with problems such as damp can directly cause ill health. And it can also be difficult to afford to heat draughty homes. As we have seen, poor families cannot afford to eat healthy foods and they may also be unable to buy safety equipment such as stair gates and fire guards. They may live in areas where there is traffic and poor street lighting and where there are few safe play areas. All of these factors can lead to poor health, accidents and even death. They can also cause stress and depression and poor mental health.

The results of all this are stark: children from poorer families are more likely to suffer respiratory infections and diseases, ear infections, squints and short stature (Blackburn 1991). According to Reid (1998), the death rates for babies (between one month and one year old) are twice as high for babies in social class V (unskilled occupations and economic inactivity, such as lone parenthood) as they are for those in social class I (professionals). This class difference in death rates remains as great for children aged between 1–5 years and 1–15 years. Differences in death rates are particularly wide for boys rather than girls. If we look at the causes of death for boys aged 1–15, the biggest differences in death rates between social classes I and V are for: accidents, fire and flame; motor accidents; and infections/parasitic diseases (Reid 1998). Class differentials in mortality rates persist into adulthood leading to wide differences in life expectancy. Men in social classes I and II (professionals and intermediate occupations) can expect to live 5 years longer than men in social classes IV and V (semi- and unskilled manual occupations).

The message here is both clear and stark: poverty not only causes ill health, it kills. It kills poor children and it kills poor adults.

9.2 Housing lone parents: tenure, ghettoisation and quality

Quality of housing both reflects a family's access to financial resources and represents an important component of living standards. For that reason, it is important to consider it in its own right. Changes in access to housing tenure of the 1980s have also reflected wider trends in increasing inequality, and in geographical concentrations of some groups. We discuss these issues below.

Council housing: an incentive to become a lone parent?

During the 1980s and early 1990s, it became common for right wing politicians (such as Peter Lilley when he was Secretary of State for Social Security and speaking to the Conservative Party Conference in 1992) to claim that single women were having babies so that they could get council accommodation (as well as access to social security in their own right). It was argued that single women knew that they would get priority for housing if they were pregnant or had a baby. They therefore deliberately get pregnant. A number of studies set out to explore whether or not this was the case and no evidence was found to support it. Rowlingson and McKay (1998) found that it was common for single women to get pregnant by accident (as do many married women). It was only once single women were pregnant that they began to make decisions about their pregnancy and looked into their housing rights, and other potential benefits.

Research with teenage mothers by Allen and Bourke-Dowling (1998) also showed that young single women do not 'play the system'. Quite the contrary, there is: 'lack of knowledge, long waits on local authority housing lists and an inability to understand the system, let alone manipulate it. We found many examples of lonely and isolated women in unsatisfactory and unsuitable . . . accommodation' (Allen and Bourke-Dowling 1998: p. 199). Nevertheless the idea of young women playing the system is a widespread one. Some teenage mothers themselves believe that other young women get pregnant for council flats. Others, however, laugh at the thought that anyone might go through pregnancy, birth and temporary accommodation just to get council accommodation. One young woman was quoted as being highly sceptical of the views of right wingers: 'They make it sound like the council put you in palaces but they don't . . . who'd want to get pregnant for the sake of being put in a council flat?' (Allen and Bourke-Dowling 1998: p. 199).

Another study by Speak *et al.* (1995) found that young mothers faced considerable difficulties in establishing an independent home. Many had limited support from their family and had to approach a number of agencies for help. Many were dissatisfied with the accommodation they had, primarily because of the nature of the neighbourhood rather than because of the quality of the accommodation. One of the greatest difficulties, however, was in being able to afford to furnish a new home. The study calculated that the cost of furnishing a home to the most basic standard from second-hand shops (without even a carpet) would cost £640. But six out of the eight lone parents who were given social fund loans were given less than £500 and a further ten were turned down for loans. Some women did not even apply for a loan because they were worried about being unable to repay it. The cost of preparing for a baby, such as a cot, bedding, clothing, pushchair or pram was also far more than level of any available state support.

While the evidence strongly disputes the view that all or most single women deliberately plan to have babies so that they can take advantage of social security and social housing, it is interesting to consider why such a suggestion causes so much moral outrage. The reason perhaps relates to a view that people should not deliberately cause themselves to be dependent on the state. Dependency on the labour market or on other individuals (in particular, husbands) is quite acceptable but dependence on the state is not. This refers us back to discussions about the underclass and also to the question posed by Jencks and Edin (1995) (discussed in Chapter 4): 'Do poor women have the right to bear children?'

Housing tenure, 'ghettoisation' and quality

During the 1980s and early 1990s, the size of the stock of council housing was reduced through restrictions on the building of new council accommodation and the 'right to buy' legislation which resulted in many council houses (particularly the most attractive properties) being sold off. This meant that only the poorest groups, such as lone parent families, remained in council accommodation. It has also been argued that certain estates have been semi-formally designated as lone parent estates, effectively ghettoising lone mothers and their children. This also raises concerns, over-played in the underclass debate, about the lack of adult male role models for children. The poor quality of the accommodation also compounds the disadvantage of this group; for example, it is likely to have an impact on the health of lone mothers and their children.

In 1999, nearly two-thirds of lone parents were social or private tenants (Marsh *et al.* 2001). This was much higher than the corresponding figure for low-income families with children (at 40 per cent). And it is twice as high as the corresponding figure for all households in England (31 per cent according to the English House Conditions Survey). Among lone parents, more than three-quarters of those out of work (78 per cent) were tenants. Housing tenure was therefore a clear indicator of social disadvantage, with a steep gradient from non-workers at one end to high-income workers at the other end (see Figure 9.1). And it was much more likely that single lone mothers and mothers separated from a cohabitation were tenants. Widows, lone fathers and previously married lone mothers were less likely to be tenants.

Lone parents are therefore more likely than average to live in social housing. And some lived in temporary accommodation. Sixteen per cent of lone parents said that they had stayed in temporary accommodation at some point and almost half of these had remained in this accommodation for longer than six months (Marsh *et al.* 2001).

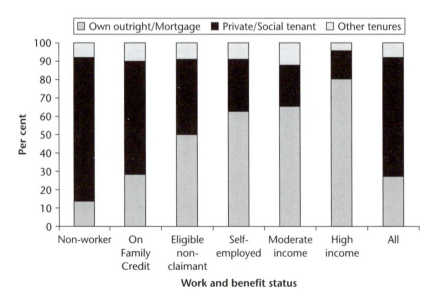

Figure 9.1 Housing tenure of lone parents by work and benefit status.
Source: Marsh *et al.* (2001: Table 2.18)

Table 9.1 Housing problems reported by lone parents in 1999

	Per cent
Problems with housing	
Rot and decay	14
Bad condensation	13
Rising damp	11
Water getting in	11
Infestations of insects	8
Plumbing	7
Electrical wiring	6
Infestations of rodents	3
Other	3
Number of problems	
None	57
1	24
2	11
3 or more	8

Source: Marsh et al. (2001: Table 6.14)

Housing *quality* is a key issue related to health, quality of life and living standards. Forty-three per cent of lone parents in 1999 reported one or more problems with their accommodation ranging from rising damp through to infestations of insects and/or rodents (see Table 9.1). Lone parents living in social housing, and those out of work, were most likely to have problems. Some had only just reported them and so had not yet had them dealt with. Others were waiting for the landlord to carry out repairs. About a quarter said that they could not deal with the problem because of lack of money.

Most of us have grown accustomed to having a central heating system but 15 per cent of lone parent families lacked this basic amenity and more than one in five of those that had central heating said that they could not keep their homes warm enough. This was partly because of the cost of doing so but also because of inefficient heating systems and poor insulation.

Overall, 15 per cent of lone parents were living in over-crowded conditions according to the 'bedroom standard' – a commonly used measure of the number of rooms each family requires (see Box 9.2). This compared with only 3 per cent of households nationally (according to the 1996 English House Conditions Survey). Rates of over-crowding were highest among non-workers and the self-employed (at 17 per cent and 21 per cent respectively). Those on high incomes were no more likely than the national average to be over-crowded.

Box 9.2   Measuring over-crowding through the 'bedroom standard'

A common way of measuring over-crowding is to apply the 'bedroom standard'. This allocates separate bedrooms to:

- each couple;
- any other person aged 21 or over;
- each pair of 10–20-year-olds of the same sex;
- each pair of 0–10-year-olds.

Unpaired people are allocated a bedroom each. This bedroom standard is then compared with the actual number of bedrooms to see whether a house is equal to, the same as, or above, the bedroom standard. However, this measure takes no account of bedroom size and some bedrooms may not be big enough for two (especially older) children to share. It may, therefore, underestimate over-crowding.

As well as being concentrated in particular tenure types, lone parents are also quite likely to be concentrated in particular places. Robertson (1984) found that lone parents in Glasgow were concentrated in the peripheral estates. Lone parents made up 16 per cent of households in periphery estates compared with 5 per cent of households in inner city areas and 2 per cent in the owner-occupied west end of the city. And within the peripheral estates, lone parents were further concentrated in particular pockets. The reason for this concentration was that the least desirable homes were the ones in peripheral estates and so these were most likely to be empty when lone parents were in need of re-housing. Thus lone parents found themselves in the estates that lacked good facilities and had poor transport links to other facilities.

It can be argued that lone parents should not be concentrated in particular estates because this is akin to ghettoisation. Certain estates might become stigmatised as being full of lone parents and their children. But if these estates have high-quality accommodation, useful facilities and good transport links, then such concentration might be seen as less problematic. Indeed, lone parents could benefit from forming informal support groups with each other. Town planners and social policy researchers continue to debate the pros and cons of mixed housing as opposed to concentrating particular groups in particular areas. Whatever the outcome of this debate it is clear that good-quality housing, useful services and good transport links are important for all household types.

Lone parents appear to be concentrated in particular estates; they are also concentrated in particular parts of the country. Analysis of the 1997 Labour Force Survey finds that almost half (45 per cent) of all lone mothers live either in London or the North West (Holtermann *et al.* 1999). The North West has the highest rate of lone parenthood followed by Wales, the North and Yorkshire/Humberside. The lowest rates are found in East Anglia and the South West. If we look within regions, we find that the highest rates of lone motherhood can be found in the metropolitan areas – particularly inner London, sub-regions of Merseyside and Tyne and Wear. More than a third of inner London families (36 per cent) are headed by a lone mother compared with 21 per cent for outer London.

One problem related to the increasingly spatial concentration of lone parents is that the areas they are concentrated in are those with far fewer employment opportunities than others (e.g. parts of Liverpool and London). The late 1990s were generally an economic success. There was an increase in the number of jobs in the country leading to some commentators to talk of the problems finding suitable people for these jobs (skills shortages). However, some parts of the country, such as the inner cities of large conurbations (particularly inner-city Liverpool and London) are still suffering from a lack of labour demand (too few jobs). The problem of a skills mismatch must therefore be seen in combination with a spatial mismatch. Turok and Edge (1999) argue that government policy has so far failed to address these issue sufficiently. Rather than focusing on supply-side issues (such as improving people's motivation to work, job-seeking skills and employable skills), the government should, in their view, be considering demand-side issues such as attracting employers to areas where joblessness is high.

The link between high rates of lone parenthood and lack of labour demand causes problems for lone parents in seeking paid work. There may also be another issue here – perhaps rates of lone parenthood are high in these areas because there are fewer opportunities for men to find decently paid jobs and therefore become potential husband–father–breadwinners. Improving employment opportunities in deprived areas for both men and women could both reduce the *hardship* faced by lone parent families and may also reduce the *number* of lone parent families. It may also reduce the duration of lone parenthood. This all reinforces the point that lone parenthood is not simply a gendered phenomenon. Gender is important and we need to recognise the place of men here as well as the experiences of women. But we also need to consider the class location of men and women and how this impacts on their lives. Another important conclusion from all of this is that, as argued throughout this book, poverty can be a significant cause as well as consequence of lone parenthood.

The government has made some attempt to tackle area deprivation with its New Deal for Communities and its Area Action Zones on health, education and employment (Social Exclusion Unit 1998, 2001). But these appear to be relatively small schemes tackling the symptoms rather than the root causes of deprivation (see also Chapter 6).

9.3 Living standards of lone parent families

In Chapter 5 we discussed the issue of poverty. We return to this general theme but this time take a broader perspective on poverty by analysing the general living standards of lone parent families. Those with the lowest living standards might be classified as suffering hardship. The distinction between poverty and hardship is an important one because whereas poverty is generally measured in terms of income at a particular point of time, measures of hardship are often related to persistent poverty. People who have lived in persistent poverty and then take a job may look well-off in terms of their current income but the backlog of poverty will take some time to clear. Equally, someone who has recently been in a job but is now out of work may have the same income as someone who has been out of work for a long time but the former's living standards are likely to be rather higher than the latter's: they have been able to build up a stock of material resources that they can draw on, for a while at least.

With all this in mind, we look first at the relative material well-being of lone parent families, for example in terms of their ability to buy items such as food, clothing, leisure and consumer durables. Then we consider how well lone parents say they were managing their money.

The most up-to-date information on lone parents, and one analysing living standards in some detail, is the survey of low-income families (SOLIF) carried out by the Policy Studies Institute for the Department of Social Security. The next section summarises some of the key findings from this survey.

Relative material well-being

Lone parents in 1999 were asked about 34 items to see whether they would like to have them but could not afford them. Inability to afford such items would be considered by many to indicate some form of material deprivation. And in some cases, lack of such items might be considered

Table 9.2 Items that lone parents and general public would like to have but cannot afford

	Lone parents unable to afford (%)	General public unable to afford (%)
Food		
Cooked main meal every day	8	–
Fresh fruit on most days	17	4
Fresh vegetable on most days	17	4
Clothing		
Weatherproof coat (for each child)	9	4
Two pairs of all-weather shoes (for each child)	25	5
New, not second-hand clothes	41	5
Leisure and entertainment		
Celebration with presents at special occasions	27	2
Toys and sports gear for children	24	–
Money for outings, trips or gifts for parties	59	–
One-week holiday away from home	74	18
Consumer durables		
Video recorder	11	2
Music system	12	–
Home computer	50	15
Telephone	9	1
Car or van	34	10

Source: Marsh et al. (2001: Tables 6.1, 6.3, 6.5 and 6.7) for lone parents; Gordon et al. (2000) for general public

to indicate social exclusion. The survey looked separately at food, clothing, leisure and entertainment, and consumer durables. Rather than reporting on all the items listed by Marsh et al. (2001), we focus on the ones that might indicate the worst levels of deprivation. We also compare the answers from lone parents with results from a survey of the general public using the same (or very similar) questions (Gordon et al. 2000). In all cases, lone parents were less well off than the population in general (Table 9.2).

About one lone parent in ten said that they could not afford to provide a cooked meal every day. And 17 per cent (a much higher proportion than for the population on average) said that they could not afford fresh fruit and vegetables on most days. Good nutrition is vital to good health. It is also important in setting children up for a day's schooling. Some schools have begun 'breakfast clubs' for their pupils because too many were going without this meal and so were not adequately nourished at the beginning of the school day. In the government's Plan for the NHS, announced in July 2000, there will be provision for a piece of fruit to be given to all children in school aged four to six.

Moving on to clothing, about one lone parent in ten said that they could not afford a weatherproof coat for each child and a quarter said that they could not afford two pairs of weatherproof shoes for each child. Two in five said that they could not afford new clothes rather than second-hand ones. The same was true for only 5 per cent of the population on average.

Expenditure on leisure and entertainment may not seem to be a basic necessity in the same way that food and clothing is, but the ability to cel-ebrate special occasions such as birthdays or to go on a one-week holiday each year may be seen as a measure of how far people (and children in particular) are able to participate in society. Overall, lone parents were less able to afford these items than food and clothing, suggesting that they prioritised material resources before leisure and entertainment. But most lone parents wanted to be able to afford leisure and entertainment for them-selves and their children. For example, only 3 per cent said that they did not want or need a one-week annual holiday away from home. Despite this, 74 per cent of lone parents said that they could not afford such a holiday and 59 per cent did not have enough money to pay for outings, trips or gifts for parties. One in three could not afford to celebrate special occasions. Deprivation was much greater for non-working lone parents. Deprivation among lone parents was also much greater here than for the population on average.

When measuring deprivation, the issue of consumer durables becomes hotly contested. Do people really need a television or a video recorder or a deep freeze or a car? The answer depends on our definition of need. If our definition of need is related to the most basic survival then the answer is no. People will not die for the lack of a video or freezer. But if our definition is related to an idea of social inclusion then we would not define need in terms of mere physical survival but in terms of ability to participate in those activities considered by most to be essential. A tele-vision would certainly be considered essential today. A deep freeze may not be considered essential but an item such as this can help people save money by enabling them to buy in bulk. Similarly a car is not a basic essen-tial according to an absolutist definition but in rural areas it becomes vital and in many areas ownership of a car is the best way of getting and keep-ing paid work.

One lone parent in ten said that they could not afford a video recorder or music system. One in ten said that they could not afford a telephone compared with only 1 per cent of the general public. A third could not afford a car or van. Half said they would like but could not afford a home computer. This last figure is higher than that for low-income couple families (at 40 per cent) and much higher than that for the general public (15 per cent). The increasing emphasis on computing in education and in employment leaves children in these families at considerable disadvantage compared with children in other families.

We may debate the importance of consumer durables and entertainment but we need to remember that substantial groups of lone parents, particularly those out of work, could not afford even basic items like food and clothing. And since 1991 average material hardship scores had increased for food, clothing and leisure and entertainment, but had fallen for consumer durables. Deprivation among lone parent families is much higher than that among the population in general.

So far we have focused on material resources. Some people have financial resources such as savings to help them through difficult times. However only a third of non-working lone parents had any savings and these were, on average (using the median), only £30. Only just over a half of non-working lone parents had a current or savings account and so relied solely on the cash economy (Marsh *et al.* 2001).

Another important set of indicators of deprivation is related to debt. About two-thirds of all non-working lone parents (and just over half of all lone parents) had one or more debts. A quarter of all lone parents had three or more debts. More than one in ten had housing arrears and these were particularly common among working lone parents who were claiming Family Credit. This is of great concern for government policy as it is seeking to encourage people to take jobs by topping up their pay with Family Credit but the interaction of Family Credit with Housing Benefit (and the lack of joined-up government between the DSS and local authorities) leaves a substantial proportion of lone parents receiving Family Credit (28 per cent) with housing debts (Marsh *et al.* 2001).

As a result of material deprivation, lack of savings, poor housing and debt, lone parents worried about money a great deal. Almost half (45 per cent) said that they worried about it all or almost all of the time (rising to 52 per cent for non-working lone parents). And almost three in ten said that they always ran out of money before the end of the week or month (rising to a third of non-working lone parents).

Marsh *et al.* (2001) combined several indicators of hardship to produce a composite score or index. A number of important findings stemmed from this, such as:

- paid work considerably reduced rates of hardship;
- lone fathers and widows experienced lower levels of hardship than average;
- single lone mothers and those separated from cohabitation suffered the highest levels of hardship;
- hardship was greater among social or private tenants than among owner-occupiers or home-owners;
- hardship increased the larger the family or the younger the children;
- lone parents with qualifications and/or a driving licence were less likely to suffer hardship;
- lone parents from ethnic minority groups suffered higher rates of hardship;
- those with health problems were more likely to suffer hardship.

9.4 Summary

Lone parents (and their children) have relatively poor levels of health and high levels of disability. They also live in poor housing. These factors, combined with their low levels of income, contribute to making this group among the most multipally-disadvantaged in the country.

In 1999, three lone parents in ten had a long-standing health problem and such problems were more common among non-workers than workers. One-third of all lone parents have at least one child with a long-term illness or disability (most commonly a respiratory disease such as asthma). Research suggests that the proportion of lone parents with health problems grew during the 1990s.

Poor health is caused by lack of income, poor housing, poor diet, unsafe environments and lack of access to health and social facilities. The results of all this are stark: the death rates for babies in social class V are twice as high as for babies in social class I. Death rates for children are similarly unequal – with the greatest disparity being between boys in terms of accidents and infectious/parasitic diseases.

Poor housing is one of the causes of poor health and a significant proportion of lone parents face problems with their accommodation, ranging from rot and decay, condensation and rising damp to infestations of insects and rodents. Most lone parent families have central heating but some do not and even those that have this facility cannot always afford to use it. Almost one non-working lone parent in every five lives in over-crowded conditions.

About two-thirds of lone parents in 1999 lived in social housing (twice the national average). Housing tenure varied considerably by type of lone parent.

It is sometimes argued that women become lone parents precisely because of the opportunity to get social housing and social security benefits. Research challenges this idea but it cannot be denied that, once single women become pregnant or once married women consider leaving a partner, the existence of social housing and social security make their final decisions to become lone parents possible. Thus social housing and social security facilitate but do not encourage lone parenthood.

The combination of low income, poor health and poor housing can result in multiple deprivation or hardship. This means that many lone parents cannot afford to buy basic items that most of us consider to be essential to modern-day life.

Material resources are part of the picture but so are financial resources such as savings. Lone parents have very few savings to help them out in a rainy day. On the contrary, in 1999, two thirds of non-working lone parents were in debt. A quarter of all lone parents had three or more debts. As a result of material deprivation, lack of savings, poor housing and debt, lone parents worried about money a great deal. Almost half said that they worried about it almost all the time.

chapter 10

Conclusions

Lone parents in Britain face an almost impossible task. Those without paid jobs have to work hard to stretch out their inadequate income to make ends meet. Those in paid work have to struggle with the conflicting demands of work and family life, usually on low incomes. Women, particularly those from poor, working class backgrounds, are expected to depend on men for the bulk of their income or, failing this, they are expected to be dependent on an employer. Those who either choose, or find themselves, outside this field of dependency, receive minimal help to survive. Those in paid work fare slightly better but their concentration in low-paid jobs still makes their lives difficult. There are some signs that, at the turn of the twenty-first century, this is changing, with increasing benefits paid to non-working lone parents, but there is still a long way to go before such benefits remove lone parent families from poverty.

Comparisons with other countries show that the link between lone parenthood and poverty need not necessarily exist. Countries where men and women, and different classes and income groups, are more equal tend not to have a high proportion of lone parents in poverty.

The main theme of this book is that the relationship between the British state and lone parent families should be understood from both a gender and class perspective. Lone parents have been a concern to the British state because they are mostly women from poor, working class backgrounds who are neither dependent on men nor the labour market (though, arguably, dependent on the state). Their children have been a concern because they are working class young people, a group that has long caused anxiety if not fear among the ruling elites. Non-resident parents have also been a concern from this perspective as they are often poor men, some of whom are outside of the apparently stabilising framework of a nuclear family. A patriarchal/capitalist state would ideally wish to see stable breadwinner/housewife nuclear families providing workers who are willing to conform to the needs of the labour market. Lone parent families challenge this picture.

While patriarchal and capitalist interests have been important for some time, other forces are also in evidence. From 1997 onwards, a Labour government, with a Minister for Women and its pledge to eradicate child poverty, is shifting the state in a new direction. It is too early, however, to see how far this will change the lives of lone parents and their families.

These conclusions draw out some of the key themes, findings and arguments presented throughout the book. These are as follows.

Lone parenthood should be seen from both a class and gender perspective (see Chapter 3)

It has become widely accepted that lone parenthood should be understood from a gender perspective. Thus it is argued that lone parents are poor because they are women. This is largely due to women's general disadvantage in relation to the labour market and the social security system. We argue that gender is clearly an important factor in relation to lone parenthood but that other factors, most particularly social class, are also important.

Lone parenthood is only a new phenomenon in comparison with earlier parts of the twentieth century (see Chapter 2)

It is probably the 1950s, and early 1960s, that stand out as unusual historically with stable families and secure male employment. However, if we take a longer look in history we find that, prior to industrialisation, lone parenthood and cohabitation were much more common than in the middle of the twentieth century. During the first half of the twentieth century, lone parenthood was less common, but there were rather more widows (such as after the two world wars, and through lower life expectancy). The last 30 years of the twentieth century saw a dramatic rise in the number of lone parents and this has concerned some commentators who bemoan the 'death of the family'.

The recent rise in lone parenthood is linked to the rise of post-industrial society (see Chapter 2)

The growth of lone parenthood, and related changes such as the growth of cohabitation, should be seen in the context of post-industrialisation. Post-industrial societies are characterised by greater flexibility in both economic and family life. These societies are moving away from the 'job for life' and 'marriage for life' model that came to dominate industrial Britain. The rise of lone parenthood is therefore related to changes in the basic structure of social and economic life. But it is also related to changes in the way that people, women in particular, choose to live their lives. Changes in people's attitudes to sex, marriage and parenthood have all contributed to the growth of lone parenthood. The relationship between socio-economic change and cultural/attitudinal change is a hotly debated subject. Whatever the precise relationship, it is clear that both factors are crucially important to the growth of lone parenthood.

Lone parents in Britain today are a diverse and dynamic group (see Chapters 1 and 9)

There is great diversity among lone parents in terms of how they became lone parents, how old they are, their health, their ethnicity and so on. Most lone parents are women from working class backgrounds but important minorities are men and people from middle class backgrounds. Lone parenthood is not usually for life. About half of all lone parents stop being lone parents within 6 years.

There is no (strong) evidence that children do worse solely as a result of living in a lone parent family (see Chapter 7)

There is much heated debate about whether or not children do worse in lone parent families. This question is incredibly difficult to answer with any confidence. The research that has been carried out suggests that, once poverty is taken into account, there is little, if any, independent effect of lone parenthood on outcomes for children. However, this is an area of both considerable controversy, and methodological difficulty.

The evidence suggests that lack of money and conflict between parents are the two key sources of problems for children. Sometimes conflict (and any violence) is reduced when couples separate but sometimes conflict (for example over child support and contact) can increase. Most of the research, however, has investigated the effects of lone parenthood through separation/divorce. There have been few studies focusing specifically on single lone parenthood. The methodological problems here are likely to be even greater as single lone parents are even poorer on average than all lone parents. So it would be very difficult to control for poverty.

Lone parenthood in Britain is strongly correlated with poverty (see Chapters 1, 5 and 9)

By any definition, most parents and children in lone parent families are poor. Too many lone parents and their children suffer poor health and live in poor housing. Hardship is rife among lone parent families.

Poverty is usually the result of lone parenthood and often the cause (see Chapters 1, 5 and 9)

Numerous studies have found that poverty is a consequence of becoming a lone parent in Britain. This is because lone parents have low rates of employment and benefit rates are relatively low. But we have to ask ourselves why benefit rates are so low and why employment rates are also low. The answer to the first question is that the state (and the taxpayers within it) do not seem prepared to ensure that lone parents and their children receive an adequate income. The answer to the second question is a complex one but one of the key issues here is that many lone mothers (like mothers in couples) see their main role in life as their children's carer. They do not see themselves as 'workers'. But many other factors are also important including childcare and financial incentives to work.

So poverty is a consequence of lone parenthood. It is also a cause of lone parenthood, particularly for single lone mothers. Lack of opportunities and 'marriageable' men is part of the explanation for why some single pregnant women decide to carry on with their pregnancies and not live with a partner.

Lone parenthood does not have to lead to poverty (see Chapter 1)

Britain has a high rate of lone parenthood, a high rate of lone parent poverty and a low rate of lone parent employment. Some other countries have similarly high rates of lone parenthood but without the corresponding problem of poverty. The Netherlands, for example, provides sufficient support for lone parents to remain in the home to look after their children without suffering poverty. Employment rates are therefore relatively low but poverty is not high. Sweden also provides relatively generous benefit payments to lone parents not in employment but it also encourages lone parents to get paid jobs. Wages are relatively high and the state provides generous childcare help so that women in paid work avoid poverty. These examples show that lone parenthood need not be synonymous with poverty. It is possible for lone parents to remain at home with their children and avoid poverty (as in the Dutch model) or to engage with the labour market and avoid poverty (as in the Swedish model). However, one of the explanations for the success of these countries is their overall level of class and gender equality. Greater equality is a fundamental prerequisite to reducing lone parent poverty.

After a slow start, the 1997 Labour government is making serious efforts to reduce child poverty

The Labour government is committed to ending child poverty. It seeks to do this using a number of measures, including: making work pay; the New Deal; childcare reforms; increases in benefits; and so on. Nevertheless, it has had to work hard following its early decision to withdraw the only benefits paid specifically to lone parents.

The main approach to reducing poverty in lone parent families is through increasing employment rates (see Chapter 6)

Employment is currently seen by the government as the best route out of poverty for lone parents. At the moment, Britain is relatively unique in not requiring much of lone parents who receive social assistance. Unlike most other countries, there is no requirement to be actively seeking work until their children are older than the school leaving age. This allows lone parents to decide for themselves about returning to work but it has also meant that those lone parents who wished to go back to work received very little help or encouragement to do so. The New Deal for Lone Parents has changed this and the forthcoming ONE system will mean that all lone parents (apart from those with pre-school-aged children) are asked to consider employment.

The move towards encouraging lone parents to take paid work could be seen as challenging the value of the unpaid 'mothering' work that women do or it could be seen as challenging women's confinement to the domestic sphere.

In general, it is better for children if lone parents have paid work

Research suggests that it is generally better for children if lone parents take up paid work. This is because it raises living standards. Having said this, low-paid work is rife among lone parent families and, despite the best efforts of in-work benefits, some working lone parents still face some hardship. But hardship levels are lower than for those with no paid work. Also, there is no evidence that children suffer emotionally from their mothers going out to work. As long as they receive suitable childcare from another source, there are no harmful effects. It is therefore important to ensure that the childcare provided is of a suitable standard.

The state's interest in non-resident parents has almost solely been in terms of their financial obligations. Their caring role has been ignored (see Chapters 7 and 8)

Non-resident fathers have received a great deal of attention from the state and the media in recent years. But it has nearly all been in relation to their financial obligations. Research generally shows a relatively low level of child support provided by non-resident parents. This is partly because they are a relatively poor group and cannot afford to pay much. It is also because they see payment of maintenance as a conditional obligation and the conditions relate to the relationship with the mother and contact with the children.

The state and media show little interest in non-resident parents' caring roles. If more attention could be paid to encouraging good parenting by non-resident parents this could help both children and lone parents within lone parent families. However, it cannot be denied that some non-resident parents might not be interested or capable of playing such a role (for example, given levels of domestic violence). But the state could, at least, consider ways of encouraging positive relationships between lone parents, non-resident parents and their children.

Children's rights are an important part of the debate on lone parenthood (see Chapters 3 and 7)

Children's rights became a key theme in the 1990s. Rather than being seen as the property of their parents, children became seen as having rights of their own. In the past, children were expected to be 'seen but not heard' and to a large extent this was reflected in research – very few studies involved talking directly to children. This is changing now with more child-centred research studies being conducted. And the power of children as consumers (the rather derogatorily labelled 'pester power') means that some children's voices are heard by parents in some circumstances.

But it still seems that children's rights are relatively weak, when the best the state is prepared to do is prevent serious harm rather than ensure a positively good quality of upbringing for children. As mentioned above, the state seeks to force non-resident parents to pay maintenance but does little even to encourage these parents to provide care and love for their children. The state is more concerned with the interests of tax-payers than the interests of children. However, the commitment to end child poverty does place children more firmly into the centre of the debate around lone parenthood so perhaps the balance between the power of the tax-payer and the child is changing very slightly.

Sources of quantitative data on lone parent families

Population censuses

The 1991 Census provides our best estimate for the number of lone parent families in Britain (Haskey 1994). Having said this, the estimates contain some uncertainty because the Census did not ask questions about the relationships between all members of each household. Estimates are therefore checked against estimates from other sources such as the General Household Survey, a continuous survey of the general. The Census is the best source of data for analysis of regional and local variation because it covers all households rather than just a sample. The 2001 Census has, at the time of going to press, just taken place. Data are likely to be available in 2003.

Bradshaw and Millar survey 1989

Sponsored by the Department of Social Security, Bradshaw and Millar carried out the first cross-sectional survey of lone parents in Britain in 1989. It had a sample of 1,428 lone parents. Lone fathers were included but widows and widowers were excluded. The sample was drawn from One Parent Benefit and Income Support records. The survey covered all aspects of life as a lone parent including income and living standards, receipt of maintenance, contact with the non-resident parent, employment, earnings, childcare and housing. Data were also collected about how people became lone parents and how they felt about being lone parents. There was an additional sample of people who had recently stopped claiming Income Support as a lone parent. These people were asked about their reasons for stopping their claim.

Policy Studies Institute surveys 1991–99

From 1991 onwards, the Department of Social Security has sponsored the Policy Studies Institute to carry out a series of surveys of lone parent families and low-income couple families. The 1991 survey was designed to evaluate the effectiveness of Family Credit, which had been introduced in 1988 but the survey also investigated broader issues relating to social security, poverty and employment. The main results from this survey were published in Marsh and McKay (1993) and McKay and Marsh (1994).

Following on from the original 1991 cross-section survey, further cross-sections of lone parents were interviewed in 1993 and 1994, and follow-up interviews with the 1991 lone parents were carried out in 1993, 1994, 1995, 1996 and 1998.

The most recent data from this set of surveys is the 1999 Survey of Low-Income Families (SOLIF), a survey including 2,800 lone parents. The sample size for this survey was much larger than for the previous studies but like the former surveys, it used Child Benefit records to sample a complete cross-section of lone parent families. Our analysis concentrates on these families but the SOLIF data also include information on low- and middle-income couple families in the bottom 40 per cent of the income distribution of families.

British Household Panel Survey (BHPS) 1994–

The BHPS was started in 1991 with a random sample of 5,500 British households containing about 10,000 people (Buck *et al.* 1994, Berthoud and Gershuny 2000). These people are re-interviewed each year along with any new partners that they live with and any children that reach the age of 16. This is not a survey specifically of lone parent families but by 1995, there were 117 mothers and 116 fathers who had experienced separation from a partner. In 1992, complete history data on previous marriages and cohabitations were collected and this has been used to study past and pre-sent spells of lone parenthood (see for example, Böheim and Ermisch 1998, Ermisch and Francesconi 1996).

National Child Development Study (NCDS)

NCDS is a series of surveys of all 17,000 babies born in Britain in one week in 1958. Data on all aspects of personal, social and economic circumstances were collected from parents and others when these children were aged 7, 11 and 16. The people themselves were interviewed at the ages of 23 and 33 and most recently in 2000 when they were 42 years old. In 1991, 23 per cent of the women remaining in the survey who had ever had children (and about 2 per cent of the fathers) had been lone parents at some point; and 10 per cent of mothers were currently lone mothers (Payne and Range 1998). The study has been used to look at outcomes for children of lone parents (e.g. Ferri 1976, 1993, Joshi and Paci 1998, Kiernan 1992, 1997). NCDS is very different from cross-sectional samples as all the people in the study are the same age. This makes comparisons between NCDS and different studies rather difficult.

Social Change and Economic Life Initiative (SCELI) 1986

This survey was located in six travel-to-work areas, and was conducted in 1986 (with a follow-up of some respondents in 1987). Respondents were aged from 20 to 60, and the survey collected complete employment, marital and child histories. Sample size was just over 6,000.

Family and Working Lives Survey (FWLS) 1994–95

This survey was similar to the Women and Employment Survey (WES) of 1980. Both these surveys interviewed a nationally representative sample (of women in WES and both men and women in FWLS). Full life and work histories were collected in both surveys making it possible to look at spells of lone parenthood. A total of 9,139 people were interviewed, aged from 16 to 69.

Labour Force Survey (LFS)

The LFS is a large-scale sample survey of the general public, carried out throughout the European Union using comparable questions and definitions. It was originally carried out each year but since 1992 it has been carried out quarterly in the UK. The sample size is huge – at 60,000 households each quarter of the year. It has been most helpfully used to look at lone parenthood, employment and ethnicity (Bartholomew *et al.* 1992, Holtermann *et al.* 1999).

Survey of non-resident fathers 1996

A total of 619 non-resident fathers were interviewed in 1996. The study was sponsored by the ESRC and found its sample of non-resident

Useful Internet sites

Government websites

Child Support Agency   http://www.dss.gov.uk/csa/

Department for Education and Skills
                    http://www.dfes.gov.uk

Department for Work and Pensions (formerly the DSS)
                    http://www.dwp.gov.uk

Inland Revenue   http://www.inlandrevenue.gov.uk/home.htm

Lord Chancellor's Department
                    http://www.open.gov.uk/lcd/

Social Exclusion Unit   http://www.cabinet-office.gov.uk/seu/

Pressure groups

CPAG   http://www.cpag.org.uk
Child Poverty Action Group

Gingerbread   http://www.gingerbread.org.uk
This site is mostly geared towards the needs of Gingerbread's members but
there is some useful information here for general browsers.

Families Need Fathers   http://www.fnf.org.uk
This is an excellent site with guides to the law relating to fatherhood as
well as summaries of recent research. It also has a very useful 'links' section

to UK government sites, advice groups, research organisations and overseas sites.

National Association for Child Support Action
                              http://www.crosswinds.net/~nacsa/
Useful links to other campaigning groups.

National Council for One Parent Families
                              http://www.oneparentfamilies.org.uk
A useful site with a series of 'factfiles' on different aspects of lone parenthood.

Research and policy organisations

Joseph Rowntree Foundation
                              http://www.jrf.org.uk
Useful 'Findings' section on this site, giving summaries of JRF-funded research.

CASE   http://sticerd.lse.ac.uk/Case/
The Centre for the Analysis of Social Exclusion, based at the London School of Economics.

IFS   http://www.ifs.org.uk/
The Institute for Fiscal Studies, an economics-based research unit specialising in tax and benefits research.

National Family and Parenting Unit
                              http://www.nfpi.org.uk/
Contains useful sections on research and policy. Also, excellent links to sites relating to parenthood in general.

One plus One   http://www.oneplusone.org.uk/

Policy Studies Institute   http://www.psi.org.uk/

Karen Rowlingson   http://www.bath.ac.uk/~ssskr/
Karen's research and teaching website.

Abbot, M. (1993) *Family Ties: English Families 1540–1920*. London: Routledge.

Acheson, D. (1998) *Inequalities in Health*. London: The Stationery Office.

Alcock, P. (1987) *Poverty and State Support*. Harlow: Longman.

Alcock, P. (1993) *Understanding Poverty*. Basingstoke: Macmillan.

Allen, I. and Bourke-Dowling, S. (1998) *Teenage Mothers*. London: Policy Studies Institute.

American Research Council (1989) *The American Family under Siege*. Washington DC: American Research Council.

Barnes, H., Day, P. and Cronin, H. (1998) *Trial and Error: A Review of UK Child Support Policy*. London: Family Policy Studies Centre.

Barrett, M. (1980) *Women's Oppression Today: Problems in Marxist Feminist Analysis*. London: Verso.

Barrett, M. and Phillips, A. (1992) *Destabilising Theory*. Cambridge: Polity.

Bartholomew, R., Hibbet, A. and Sidaway, J. (1992) 'Lone parent families and the labour market: evidence from the Labour Force Survey', *Employment Gazette*, London: Employment Department, November.

Bauman, Z. (1992) *Intimations of Postmodernity*. London: Routledge.

Beck, U. and Beck-Gernsheim, E. (1995) *The Normal Chaos of Love*. Cambridge: Polity Press.

Beishon, S., Modood, T. and Virdee, S. (1998) *Ethnic Minority Families*. London: Policy Studies Institute.

Berthoud, R. (2000) 'Family formation in multi-cultural Britain: three patterns of diversity', Institute for Social and Economic Research, Research Working Paper 34. Essex: University of Essex.

Berthoud, R. (2001) 'Teenage births to ethnic minority women', in *Population Trends* (forthcoming).

Berthoud, R. and Ford, R. (1996) *Relative Needs: Variations in the Living Standards of Different Types of Households*. London: Policy Studies Institute.

Berthoud, R. and Gershuny, J. (eds) (2000) *Seven Years in the Lives of British Families*. Bristol: Policy Press.

Bieback, K. (1992) 'Family Benefits in Australia, Germany and Britain', *Journal of European Social Policy*, 2 (4): 239–254.

Blackburn, C. (1991) *Poverty and Health: Working with Families*. Milton Keynes: Open University Press.

Blackstone, W. (1775) *Commentaries on the Laws of England*, Book 1, 7th edition. Oxford: Clarendon Press.

Blake, J. and Das Gupta, P. (1975) 'Reproductive motivation versus contraceptive technology: is recent American experience an exception?', *Population and Development Review*, 1: 229–249.

Böheim, R. and Ermisch, J. (1998) 'Analysis of the dynamics of lone parent families', Working Paper 98–8. Essex: ESRC Centre on Micro-social Change.

Bowlby, J. (1951) *Maternal Care and Mental Health*. Geneva: World Health Organization.

Bradley, H. (1996) *Fractured Identities: Changing Patterns of Inequality*. Cambridge: Polity Press.

Bradshaw, J. (1999) 'The nature of poverty', in Ditch, J. (ed.) *Introduction to Social Security*. London: Routledge.

Bradshaw, J. and Millar, J. (1991) *Lone parent families in the UK*. London: HMSO (DSS Research Report No. 6).

Bradshaw, J., Kennedy, S., Kilkey, M., Hutton, S., Cordon, A., Eardley, T., Holmes, H. and Neale, J. (1996) *The Employment of Lone Parents: a Comparison of Policy in 20 Countries*. London: HMSO.

Bradshaw, J., Stimson, C., Skinner, C. and Williams, J. (1999) *Absent Fathers*. London: Routledge.

Brannen, J. and O'Brien, M. (eds) (1995) *Childhood and Parenthood*. London: Institute of Education.

Brannen, J. and O'Brien, M. (eds) (1996) *Children and Families: Research and Policy*. London: Falmer Press.

Bryson, A., Ford, R. and White, M. (1997) *Making Work Pay: Lone Mothers' Employment and Well-being*. York: Joseph Rowntree Foundation.

Buck, N., Gershuny, J., Rose, N. and Scott, J. (eds) (1994) *Changing Households: the BHPS 1990–92*. Colchester: ESRC Research Centre on Micro-social Change.

Burgess, A. and Ruxton, S. (1996) *Men and their children*. London: Institute for Public Policy Research.

Burghes, L. (1994) *Lone Parenthood and Family Disruption: The Outcomes for Children*. London: Family Policy Studies Centre.

Burghes, L., Clarke, L. and Cronin, N. (1997) *Families and Fatherhood in Britain*. London: Family Policy Studies Centre.

Burgoyne, C. and Millar, J. (1994) 'Child support: the views of fathers', *Policy and Politics*, 22: 95–104.

Central Statistical Office (1996) *Living in Britain: General Household Survey 1994*. London: HMSO.

Cherlin, A. (1992) *Marriage, Divorce, Remarriage*. Cambridge, MA: Harvard University Press.

Child Poverty Action Group (1999/2000) *Welfare Benefits Handbook*, Volume 2. London: Child Poverty Action Group.

Clarke, K., Craig, G. and Glendinning, C. (1996) *Children's Views on Child Support: Parents, Families and Responsibilities*. London: Children's Society.

Cockett, M. and Tripp, J. (1994) *The Exeter Family Study: Family Breakdown and its Impact on Children*. Exeter: University of Exeter Press.

Coleman, D. and Chandola, T. (1999) 'Britain's place in Europe's population', in McRae, S. (ed.) *Changing Britain: Families and Households in the 1990s*. Oxford: Oxford University Press.

Corden, A. (1999) *Making Child Maintenance Regimes Work*. London: Family Policy Studies Centre.

Corsaro, W. (1997) *The Sociology of Childhood*. Thousand Oaks, CA: Pine Forge Press.

Crompton, R. and Sanderson, K. (1990) *Gendered Jobs and Social Change*. London: Unwin Hyman.

Crow, G. and Hardey, M. (1992) 'Diversity and ambiguity among lone parent households in modern Britain', in Marsh, C. and Arber, S. *Families and Households: Division and Change*. British Sociological Association, London: Macmillan.

Daniel, P. and Ivatts, J. (1998) *Children and Social Policy*. Basingstoke: Macmillan.

Dennis, N. and Erdos, G. (1992) *Families without Fatherhood*. London: Institute of Economic Affairs.

Department of Social Security (1990) *Children Come First*, CM 1263.

Department of Social Security (1998) *Children First: A New Approach to Child Support*, CM 3992.

Department of Social Security (2000) *Households Below Average Income 1994/5–1998/9*. London: DSS.

Department of Social Security (2000a) *Fact Sheets on Social Security*. London: DSS.

Department of Trade and Industry (2000) *Work and Parents: Competitiveness and Choice*. London: DTI, Cm 5005.

Dilnot, A. and Duncan, A. (1992) 'Lone mothers, family credit and paid work', *Fiscal Studies*, 13 (1).

Dorsett, R. and Marsh, A. (1998) *The Health Trap*. London: Policy Studies Institute.

Dowler, E. and Calvert, C. (1995) *Nutrition and Diet in Lone Parent Families in London*. London: Family Policy Studies Centre.

Duncan, S. and Edwards, R. (eds) (1997) *Single Mothers in an International Context: Mothers or Workers?* London: UCL Press.

Duncan, S. and Edwards, R. (1999) *Lone Mothers, Paid Work and Gendered Moral Rationalities*. Basingstoke: Palgrave.

Durham, M. (1991) *Sex and Politics; The Family and Morality in the Thatcher Years*. Basingstoke: Macmillan.

Eekelaar, J. (1997) *Regulating Divorce*. Oxford: Clarendon Press.

Engels, F. (1972) *The Origin of the Family, Private Property and the State*. London: Lawrence Wishart.

Ermisch, J. (1991) *Lone Parenthood: An Economic Analysis*. Cambridge: Cambridge University Press.

Eisenstein, Z. (ed.) (1979) *Capitalist Patriarchy*. New York: Monthly Review Press.

Ermisch, J. and Francesconi, M. (1996) 'The increasing complexity of family relationships: lifetime experience of single motherhood and stepfamilies in Great Britain', Working Papers of the ESRC Research Centre on Micro-social Change, Paper no. 96–11.

Ermisch, J. and Francesconi, M. (2001) *The Effects of parents' employment on children's lives*. London: Family Policy Studies Centre.

Esping-Andersen, G. (1990) *The Three Worlds of Welfare Capitalism*. Cambridge: Polity Press.

Evans, D. (1993) *Sexual Citizenship*. London: Routledge.

Ferri, E. (1976) *Growing up in a one-parent family*. Windsor: NFER.

Ferri, E. (1993) *Life at 33: the 5th follow-up of the NCDS*. London: NCB.

Field, F. (1989) *Losing Out: The Emergence of Britain's Underclass*. Oxford: Basil Blackwell.

Finer, M. (1974) *Report of the Committee on One-parent Families*, Cmnd 5629. London: HMSO.

Firestone, S. (1971) *The Dialectic of Sex*. London: Jonathan Cape.

Flandrin, J.-L. (1979) *Families in Former Times*. Cambridge: Cambridge University Press.

Ford, R. (1996) *Childcare in the Balance: How Lone Parents Make Decisions About Work*. London: PSI.

Ford, R., Marsh, A. and McKay, S. (1995) *Changes in Lone Parenthood*. DSS Research Report No. 40, London: HMSO.

Ford, R, Marsh, A. and Finlayson, L. (1998) *What Happens to Lone Parents*. DSS Research Report No. 77, London: The Stationery Office.

Fox Harding, L. (1996) *Family, State and Social Policy*. London: Macmillan.

Furstenberg, F. and Cherlin, A. (1991) *Divided Families, What Happens to Children?* Cambridge, MA: Harvard University Press.

Garfinkel, I. and McLanahan, S. (1986) *Single Mothers and their Children: A New American Dilemma*. Washington, DC: The Urban Institute Press.

Gauthier, A. (1996) *The State and the Family: A Comparative Analysis of Family Policies in Industrialised Countries*. Oxford: Clarendon Press.

Giddens, A. (1991) *Modernity and Self-identity*. Cambridge: Polity Press.

Giddens, A. (1992) *The Transformation of Intimacy*. Cambridge: Polity Press.

Gillis, J. (1985) *For Better, For Worse: British Marriages, 1600 to the present*. Oxford: Oxford University Press.

Glendinning, C. and Millar, J. (eds) (1992) *Women and Poverty in Britain: the 1990s*. Hemel Hempstead: Wheatsheaf.

Goode, J., Callender, C. and Lister, R. (1998) *Purse or Wallet? Gender Inequalities and Income Distribution Within Families on Benefit*. London: PSI.

Gordon, D., Adelman, L., Ashworth, K., Bradshaw, J., Levitas, R., Middleton, S., Pantazis, C., Patsios, D., Payne, S., Townsend, P. and Williams, J. (2000) *Poverty and Social Exclusion*. York: Joseph Rowntree Foundation.

Grace, S. (1995) *Policing Domestic Violence in the 1990s*. Home Office Research Study 139, London: Home Office Research and Planning Unit.

Gregory, J. and Foster, K. (1990) *The Consequences of Divorce: The Report of the 1984 Consequences of Divorce Survey Carried Out on Behalf of the Lord Chancellor's Department*. London: HMSO.

Grint, K. (1991) *Sociology of Work*. Oxford: Polity Press.

Gummer, J. (1971) *The Permissive Society: The Guardian Enquiry*. London: Panther.

Hakim, C. (1991) 'Grateful slaves and self-made women: fact and fantasy in women's work orientation', *European Sociological Review*, 7/2: 101–121.

Hales, J., Lessof, C., Roth, W., Gloyer, M., Shaw, A. Millar, J., Barnes, M., Elias, P., Hasluck, C., McKnight, A. and Green, A. (2000a) *Evaluation of the New Deal for Lone Parents: Early Lessons from the Phase One Prototype – Synthesis Report*. DSS Research Report No. 108, Leeds: Corporate Document Services.

Hales, J., Roth, W., Barnes, M., Millar, J., Lessof, C., Gloyer, M. and Shaw, A. (2000b) *Evaluation of the New Deal for Lone Parents: Early Lessons from the Phase One Prototype – Findings of Surveys*. DSS Research Report No. 109, Leeds: Corporate Document Services.

Harrison, S. (1996) 'Piggy in the middle: what happens to you when your parents separate', in Long, M. (ed.) *Children in Charge: The Child's Right to a Fair Hearing*. London: Jessica Kingsley.

Haskey, J. (1994) 'Estimated numbers of one-parent families and their prevalence in Great Britain in 1991', *Population Trends*, 78: 5–19.

Haskey, J. (1998) 'One-parent families and their dependent children in Great Britain', in Ford, R. and Millar, J. (eds) *Private Lives and Public Responses: Lone Parenthood and the Future of Policy in the UK*. London: Policy Studies Institute.

Heath, A. (1992) 'The attitudes of the underclass', in Smith, D. (ed.) *Understanding the Underclass*. London: Policy Studies Institute.

Hibbert, C. (1987) *The English: A Social History 1066–1945*. London: Guild Publishing.

Hill, M. and Tisdall, K. (1997) *Children and Society*. Harlow: Longman.

Hills, J. (1995) *Inquiry into Income and Wealth: volume 2*. York: Joseph Rowntree Foundation.

Hirsch, D. (2000) *A Credit to Children: The UK's Radical Reform of Children's Benefits in an International Perspective*. York: Joseph Rowntree Foundation.

HM Treasury (2000) *The Modernization of Britain's Tax and Benefit System, Number 6*. London: HM Treasury.

Hobcraft, J. and Kiernan, K. (1999) *Childhood Poverty, Early Motherhood and Adult Social Exclusion*. CASE paper 28, London: LSE.

Holtermann, S., Brannen, J., Moss, P. and Owen, C. (1999) *Lone Parents and the Labour Market: Results from the 1997 Labour Force Survey and Review of Research*. London: Employment Service Report 23.

Home Office (1998) *Supporting Families*. London: Home Office.

Hooper, C. (1994) 'Do families need fathers? The impact of divorce on children', in Mullender, A. and Morley, R. (eds) *Children Living with Domestic Violence*. Bournemouth: Bourne Press.

Houghton-James, H. (1994) 'Children divorcing their parents', *Social Welfare and Family Law*, 6: 221.

Houlbrooke, R. (1984) *The English Family*. London: Longman.

House of Commons, HC 798 (1999) *The 1999 Child Support White Paper*, Social Security Committee Tenth Report, Session 1998–1999. London: The Stationery Office.

Hoynes, H. (1996) *Work, Welfare and Family Structure: A Review of the Evidence*. Institute for Research on Poverty, Discussion Paper No. 1, 103–196, Madison, WI: University of Wisconsin.

Ingelhart, R. (1977) *The Silent Revolution: Changing Values and Political Styles among Western Publics*. Princeton, NJ: Princeton University Press.

Ingelhart, R. (1990) *Culture Shift in Advanced Industrial Society*. Princeton, NJ: Princeton University Press.

Inland Revenue (2001) *WFTC Statistics*. London: Inland Revenue.

James, A. (1999) 'Parents: a child's perspective', in Bainham, A., Sclater, S. and Richards, M. *What is a Parent? A Socio-legal Analysis*. Oxford: Hart Publishing.

Jencks, C. and Edin, K. (1995) 'Do poor women have a right to bear children?', *The American Prospect*, 20: 43–52.

Joshi, H. and Paci, P. (1998) *Unequal Pay for Men and Women*, Cambridge, MA: Mass. Institution of Technology Press.

Kamerman, S. and Kahn, A. (eds) (1978) *Family Policy: Government and Family in 14 Countries*. New York: Columbia University Press.

Kamerman, S. and Kahn, A. (eds) (1997) *Family Change and Family Policies in Great Britain, Canada, New Zealand and the United States*. Oxford: Clarendon Press.

Kempson, E. (1996) *Life on a Low Income*. York: Joseph Rowntree Foundation.

Kempson, E., Bryson, A. and Rowlingson, K. (1994) *Hard Times? How Poor Families Make Ends Meet*. London: Policy Studies Institute.

Kiernan, K. (1992) 'Men and women at work and at home', in Jowell, R., Brook, L., Prior, G. and Taylor, B. *British Social Attitudes, 9th report*. London: SCPR.

Kiernan, K. (1996) 'Lone parents, employment and outcomes for children', *International Journal of Law, Policy and the Family*, 10: 233–249.

Kiernan, K. (1997) *The Legacy of Parental Divorce*. London: Centre for Analysis of Social Exclusion.

Kiernan, K. and Wicks, M. (1990) *Family Change and Future Policy*. London: Family Policy Studies Centre.

Kiernan, K., Land, H. and Lewis, J. (1998) *Lone Motherhood in 20th Century Britain*. Oxford: Oxford University Press.

Knijn, T. and van Wel, F. (2001) 'Does it work? Employment policies for lone parents in the Netherlands', in Millar, J. and Rowlingson, K. (eds) (2001) *Lone parents, employment and social policy: cross-national comparisons*. Bristol: Policy Press (in press).

Land, H. (1994) 'Reversing the inadvertent nationalization of fatherhood: the British Child Support Act 1991 and its consequences for men, women and children', *International Social Security Review*, 3–4: 91–100.

Land, H. (2001) 'Lone mothers, employment and childcare', in Millar, J. and Rowlingson, K. (eds) *Lone Parents, Employment and Social Policy: Cross-national Comparisons*. Bristol: Policy Press (in press).

Levitas, R. (1996) 'The concept of social exclusion and the new Durkheimian hegemony', *Critical Social Policy*, 16 (1): 5–20.

Lewis, J. (1980) *The politics of motherhood*. London: Croom Helm.

Lewis, J. (1992) 'Gender and the development of welfare regimes', *Journal of European Social Policy*, 2 (3): 159–173.

Lewis, J. (2000) 'Why don't fathers pay more for their children?', *Benefits*, 27, Jan/Feb.

Lewis, J. with Hobson, B. (1997) 'Introduction', in Lewis, J. (ed.) *Lone Mothers in European Welfare Regimes*. London: Jessica Kingsley.

Lyotard, J.-F. (1984) *The Postmodern Condition*. Manchester: Manchester University Press.

Macfarlane, A. (1986) *Marriage and Love in England 1300–1840*. Oxford: Basil Blackwell.

Mack, J. and Lansley, S. (1985) *Poor Britain*. London: Allen and Unwin.

McKay, S. and Marsh, A. (1994) *Lone Parents and Work: The Effects of Benefits and Maintenance*. London: HMSO.

McKay, S. and Rowlingson, K. (1999) *Social Security in Britain*. Basingstoke: Macmillan.

McLaren, A. (1978) *Birth Control in 19th century England*. London: Croom Helm.

McLaughlin, E. (1999) 'Social security and poverty: women's business', in Ditch, J. (ed.) *Introduction to Social Security*. London: Routledge.

Maclean, M. and Eekelaar, J. (1997) *The Parental Obligation*. Oxford: Hart Publishing.

Maclean, M. and Richards, M. (1999) 'Parents and divorce: changing patterns', in Bainham, A., Sclater, S. and Richards, M. *What is a Parent? A socio-legal analysis*. Oxford: Hart Publishing.

Marsden, D. (1969) *Mothers Alone: Poverty and the Fatherless Family*. Harmondsworth: Penguin Press.

Marsh, A. and McKay, S. (1993) *Families, Work and Benefits*. London: Policy Studies Institute.

Marsh, A. and McKay, S. (1994) *Poor Smokers*. London: Policy Studies Institute.

Marsh, A., McKay, S., Smith, A. and Stephenson, A. (2001) *Low-income Families in Britain: Work, Welfare and Social Security in 1999*. London: Policy Studies Institute.

Marx, K. and Engels, F. [1849] (1934) *The Communist Manifesto*. London: Lawrence and Wishart.

Mayer, S. (1997) *What Money Can't Buy: Family Income and Children's Life Chances*. Cambridge, MA: Harvard University Press.

Middleton, S., Ashworth, K. and Walker, R. (eds) (1994) *Family Fortunes*. London: Child Poverty Action Group.

Millar, J. (1992) 'Lone mothers and poverty', in Glendinning, C. and Millar, J. (eds) *Women and poverty in Britain: the 1990s*. Hemel Hempstead: Wheatsheaf.

Millar, J. (1998) 'Social policy and family policy', in Alcock, P., Erskine, A. and May, M. (eds) *The student's companion to social policy*. Oxford: Blackwell and Social Policy Association.

Millar, J. (1999) 'State, family and personal responsibility: the changing balance for lone mothers in the UK', in Allan, G. (ed.) *The sociology of the family: a reader*. Oxford: Blackwell.

Millar, J. (2001) 'Work requirements and labour market programmes for lone parents', in Millar, J. and Rowlingson, K. (eds) *Lone Parents, Employment and Social Policy: Cross-national Comparisons*. Bristol: Policy Press (in press).

Millar, J. and Glendinning, C. (1992) 'Gender divisions and poverty', in Glendinning, C. and Millar, J. (eds) *Women and poverty in Britain: the 1990s*. Hemel Hempstead: Wheatsheaf.

Millar, J. and Rowlingson, K. (eds) (2001) *Lone Parents, Employment and Social Policy: Cross-national Comparisons*. Bristol: Policy Press (in press).

Millar, J. and Whiteford, P. (1993) 'Child support in lone-parent families: policies in Australia and the UK', *Policy and Politics*, 21 (1): 59–72.

Millett, K. (1971) *Sexual Politics*. London: Sphere.

Mirrlees-Black, C. (1999) *Domestic Violence: Findings from a new British Crime Survey Self-completion Questionnaire*. Home Office Research Study 191, London: Home Office Research and Planning Unit.

Mitchell, A. (1984) *Children in the Middle*. London: Tavistock.

Morgan, P. (1995) *Farewell to the Family: Public Policy and Family Breakdown*. London: Institute of Economic Affairs.

Morley, R. and Mullender, A. (1994) 'Domestic violence and children: what do we know from the research?', in Mullender, A. and Morley, R. (eds) *Children Living with Domestic Violence*. Bournemouth: Bourne Press.

Murray, C. (1996a) 'The emerging British underclass', in Lister, R. (ed.) *Charles Murray and the Underclass: The Developing Debate*. London: Institute of Economic Affairs.

Murray, C. (1996b) 'Underclass: the crisis deepens', in Lister, R. (ed.) *Charles Murray and the Underclass: The Developing Debate*. London: Institute of Economic Affairs.

Noble, M., Smith, G. and Cheung, S. (1998) *Lone Mothers Moving in and out of Benefits*. York: Joseph Rowntree Foundation.

Office of National Statistics (2000) *Social Trends, 30*. London: The Stationery Office.

Office of National Statistics (2001) *Social Trends, 31*. London: The Stationery Office.

Oldfield, N. and Yu, A. (1993) *The Cost of a Child: Living Standards for the 1990s*. London: Child Poverty Action Group.

Orloff, A. (1993) 'Gender and the social rights of citizenship', *American Sociological Review*, 58: 303–328.

Parsons, T. (1951) *The Social System*. Glencoe, IL: Free Press.

Parsons, T. and Bales, R. (1956) *Family, Socialisations and Interaction Process*. London: Routledge and Kegan Paul.

Parton, N. (1991) *Governing the Family*. Basingstoke: Macmillan.

Payne, J. and Range, M. (1998) *Lone Parents' Lives*. London: The Stationery Office.

Pedersen, S. (1993) *Family, Dependence and the Origins of the Welfare State*. Cambridge: Cambridge University Press.

Pedersen, L., Weise, H., Jacobs, S. and White, M. (2000) 'Lone mothers' poverty and employment', in Gallie, D. and Paugum, S. (eds) *Welfare Regimes and the Experience of Unemployment*. Oxford: Oxford University Press, pp. 175–199.

Peterson, J. and Zill, N. (1986) 'Marital disruption, parent–child relationships and behavior problems in children', *Journal of Marriage and the Family*, 48: 295–307.

Phoenix, A., Woollett, A. and Lloyd, E. (eds) (1991) *Motherhood: Meanings, Practices and Ideologies*. London: Sage.

Piachaud, D. and Sutherland, H. (2000) 'How effective is the British government's attempt to reduce child poverty?', *CASE paper 38*, London: London School of Economics.

Pickford, R. (1999) 'Unmarried fathers and the law', in Bainham, A., Sclater, S. and Richards, M. *What is a parent? A socio-legal analysis*. Oxford: Hart Publishing.

Plotnikoff, J. and Woolfson, R. (1998) *Policing Domestic Violence*. Policy Research Series Paper 100, London: Home Office Research Development Statistics.

Population Trends (1999) 'Conceptions in England and Wales, 1997', 95: 47–56.

Qvortrup, J., Bardy, M., Sgritta, G. and Wintersberger, H. (eds) (1994) *Childhood Matters*. Aldershot: Avebury.

Reeves, R. (2000) 'The way we work: bias against women won't just go away', *The Guardian*, 30 August 2000.

Reid, I. (1998) *Class in Britain*. Oxford: Polity Press.

Roberts, E. (1995) *Women and Families: An Oral History*. Oxford: Blackwell.

Robertson, I. (1984) 'Single parent lifestyle and peripheral estate residence', *Town Planning Review*, 55: 197–213.

Rodgers, B. and Pryor, J. (1998) *Divorce and Separation: The Outcomes for Children*. London: Joseph Rowntree Foundation.

Rogers, W.S. and Roche, J. (1994) *Children's Welfare and Children's Rights*. London: Hodder and Stoughton.

Room, G. (ed.) (1995) *Beyond The threshold: The Measurement and Analysis of Social Exclusion*. Bristol: Policy Press.

Rowbotham, S. (1981) 'The trouble with patriarchy', in Feminist Anthology Collective (ed.) *No Turning Back*, London: Women's Press, pp. 72–78.

Rowlingson, K. and McKay, S. (1998) *The Growth of Lone Parenthood: Diversity and Dynamics*. London: Policy Studies Institute.

Rowntree, S. (1901) *Poverty: A Study of Town Life*. London: Macmillan.

Runciman, W. (1990) 'How many classes are there in contemporary British society?', *Sociology*, 24 (3).

Sainsbury, D. (1996) *Gender Equality and Welfare States*. Cambridge: Cambridge University Press.

Sawhill, I. (ed.) (1995) *Welfare Reform: an Analysis of the Issues*. Washington, DC: Urban Institute.

Searle, G. (1976) *Eugenics and Politics in Britain, 1900–1914*. Leyden: Noordhof International Publishing.

Silva, E. (ed.) (1996) *Good Enough Mothering*. London: Routledge.

Silva, E. and Smart, C. (eds) (1999) *The New Family?* London: Sage.

Skevik, A. (2001) 'Lone parents and employment in Norway', in Millar, J. and Rowlingson, K. (eds) *Lone Parents, Employment and Social Policy: Cross-national Comparisons*. Bristol: Policy Press (in press).

Skinner, C. and Bradshaw, J. (2000) 'Non-resident fathers, child support and contact', *Benefits*, 27, Jan/Feb.

Smart, C. and Neale, B. (1999) *Family Fragments?* Cambridge: Polity Press.

Smith, D. (ed.) (1992) *Understanding the Underclass*. London: Policy Studies Institute.

Snell, K. and Millar, J. (1987) 'Lone parent families and the welfare state: past and present', *Continuity and Change*, 2, part 3.

Social Exclusion Unit (1998) *Bringing Britain together: A National Strategy for Neighbourhood Renewal*. London: SEU.

Social Exclusion Unit (1999) *Teenage Pregnancy*. Cm 4342, London: SEU.

Social Exclusion Unit (2001) *A New Commitment to Neighbourhood Renewal: A National Strategy Action plan*. London: SEU.

Soloway, R. (1990) *Demography and Degeneration: Eugenics and the Declining Birthrate*. Chapel Hill, NC: University of North Carolina Press.

Song, M. and Edwards, R. (1996) 'Raising questions about perspectives on black lone motherhood', *Journal of Social Policy*, 26 (2): 233–244.

Speak, S., Cameron, S., Woods, R. and Gilroy, R. (1995) *Young Single Mothers: Barriers to Independent Living*. London: Family Policy Studies Centre.

Speed, M. and Kent, N. (1996) *Child Support National Client Satisfaction Survey 1995*. DSS Research Report No. 51, London: HMSO.

Spicker, P. (1993) *Poverty and Social Security*. London: Routledge.

Stacey, J. (1993) 'Untangling feminist theory', in Richardson, D. and Robinson, V. (eds) *Introducing Women's Studies*. London: Macmillan.

Stone, L. (1990) *The Road to Divorce*. Oxford: Oxford University Press.

Thornton, A. (1985) 'Changing attitudes towards separation and divorce: causes and consequences', *American Journal of Sociology*, 90: 856–872.

Tizard, B. (1991) 'Employed mothers and the care of young children', in Phoenix, A., Woollett, A. and Lloyd, E. (eds) *Motherhood: Meanings, Practices and Ideologies*. London: Sage.

Townsend, P. (1979) *Poverty in the United Kingdom*. Harmondsworth: Penguin.

Turok, I. and Edge, N. (1999) *The Jobs Gap in Britain's Cities*. York: Joseph Rowntree Foundation.

Veit-Wilson, J. (1999) 'Poverty and the adequacy of social security', in Ditch, J. (ed.) *Introduction to Social Security*. London: Routledge.

Vincent, A. (1987) *Theories of the State*. Oxford: Basil Blackwell.

Walby, S. (1986) *Patriarchy at Work*. Oxford: Basil Blackwell.

Waldfogel, J. (1997) 'Ending Welfare as we know it: the Personal Responsibility and Work Opportunity Act of 1996', *Benefits*, 20, Sept/Oct.

Waldfogel, J., Danziger, S.K., Danziger, S. and Seefeldt, K. (2001) 'Welfare reform and lone mothers' employment in the US', in Millar, J. and Rowlingson, K. (eds) *Lone Parents, Employment and Social Policy: Cross-national Comparisons*. Bristol: Policy Press (in press).

Wasoff, F. and Dey, I. (2000) *Family Policy*. Eastbourne: Gildredge Press.

Wellings, K., Field, J., Johnson, A. and Wadsworth, J. (1994) *Sexual Behaviour in Britain*. Harmondsworth: Penguin.

Wheen, F. (2000) 'Violence begins at home', *The Guardian*, 2 August.

White, M. (2000) *The Employment of Lone Mothers in Denmark and Great Britain*. London: DSS/ASD5: In-house Report No. 72.

Whiteford, P. and Bradshaw, J. (1994) 'Benefits and incentives for lone parents: a comparative analysis', *International Social Security Review*, 47 (3–4): 69–89.

World Health Organization Expert Committee on Mental Health (1951) *Report on the Second Session*. Geneva: WHO.

Wright, G. and Stetson, D. (1978) 'The impact of no-fault divorce law reform on divorce in American States', *Journal of Marriage and the Family*, 40: 575–580.

index